Pain

its nature
and treatment

Commissioning Editor: Michael Parkinson
Development Editor: Hannah Kenner
Project Manager: Joannah Duncan
Senior Designer: Sarah Russell
Illustrator: Hardlines

Pain

its nature and treatment

Sir Michael R. Bond

MD PhD DSc DUniv FRCS FRCPsych
FRCP FRCA FRSE FRSA

Emeritus Professor of Psychological Medicine
University of Glasgow
Glasgow, UK

Karen H. Simpson

MBCHB FRCA

Consultant in Anaesthesia and Pain Management
Pain Management Service
St James's University Hospital
Leeds, UK

Foreword by
Professor Ronald Melzack PhD FRCS
Emeritus Professor, Department of Psychology
McGill University
Montreal, Quebec, Canada

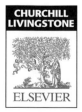

CHURCHILL
LIVINGSTONE

ELSEVIER

Edinburgh London New York Oxford Philadelphia St Louis Sydney Toronto 2006

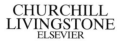

CHURCHILL LIVINGSTONE
ELSEVIER

First published 2006

ISBN 0 443 06352 4

British Library Cataloguing in Publication Data
A catalogue record for this book is available from the British Library

Library of Congress Cataloging in Publication Data
A catalog record for this book is available from the Library of Congress

Note
Medical knowledge is constantly changing. Standard safety precautions must be followed, but as new research and clinical experience broaden our knowledge, changes in treatment and drug therapy may become necessary or appropriate. Readers are advised to check the most current product information provided by the manufacturer of each drug to be administered to verify the recommended dose, the method and duration of administration, and contraindications. It is the responsibility of the practitioner, relying on experience and knowledge of the patient, to determine dosages and the best treatment for each individual patient. Neither the Publisher nor the authors assume any liability for any injury and/or damage to persons or property arising from this publication.

The Publisher

Working together to grow libraries in developing countries

www.elsevier.com | www.bookaid.org | www.sabre.org

ELSEVIER   BOOK AID International   Sabre Foundation

 ELSEVIER   your source for books, journals and multimedia in the health sciences
www.elsevierhealth.com

The Publisher's policy is to use **paper manufactured from sustainable forests**

Printed in China

Contents

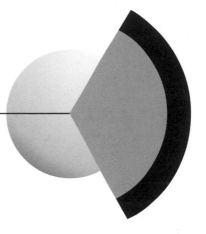

CONTENTS

Foreword

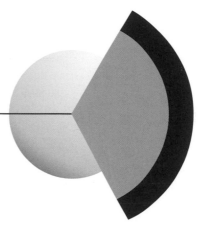

The field of pain has recently undergone a major revolution. Historically, pain is a sensation produced by injury or disease. We now possess a much broader concept of pain that includes the emotional, cognitive and sensory dimensions of pain experience, as well as an impressive array of new approaches to pain management.

By recognizing the dominant role of the brain, which creates our subjective experiences of pain and activates our neuroendocrine and immune defence systems, we are now able to appreciate the intimate relationship between pain and stress. We are so accustomed to considering pain as a purely sensory phenomenon that we have long ignored the fact that injury does more than produce pain; it also disrupts the brain's homeostatic regulation systems, thereby producing stress and initiating complex programmes to reinstate homeostasis. The stress system vastly expands the puzzle of pain and provides valuable clues in our quest to understand chronic pain. Many autoimmune diseases such as rheumatoid arthritis, lupus and scleroderma are also pain syndromes. Furthermore, more women than men suffer from these syndromes. These relationships among gender, the immune system, and chronic pain syndromes reveal the necessity to study pain in a biological context far broader than a spinal 'pain pathway' as the central focus of theory and research.

Despite the impressive advances and optimistic outlook, many chronic pains remain intractable. Consider phantom limb pain. About 60–70% of amputees suffer terrible persistent pain. The pain may be relieved in some patients by local anaesthetic injections or a combination of drugs. But, tragically, the cause of the pain is poorly understood and no widely effective treatment has yet been found. Similarly some people who suffer chronic headaches, backaches, fibromyalgia, pelvic pain and other forms of chronic pain are helped by several therapies that are now available, but most are not. For example, we have excellent new drugs for some kinds of headache, but not for all. The continued suffering by millions of people indicates we still have a long way to go.

This excellent introductory textbook by Michael Bond and Karen Simpson covers every important facet of the field of pain. It describes the rapid growth of research and theory, and the recent advances in diagnosing and managing clinical pain states. The book also presents procedures and strategies to combat a wide range of acute and chronic pains. Unfortunately, many people suffering various forms of pain are not helped because we lack the necessary knowledge. Still worse, many people suffer even though we have the knowledge but our educational, healthcare or other social systems have failed. This book is a valuable contribution to the field of pain by providing up-to-date knowledge that will stimulate a new generation of scientists and health professionals.

The ongoing pain revolution has taken us from a specific pain pathway to an open biological system that comprises multiple sensory inputs, memories of past experiences, personal and social expectations, genetic contributions, gender, aging, and stress patterns involving the endocrine, autonomic and immune systems. Pain has become a major challenge to medicine, psychology, and all the other health sciences and professions. Every aspect of life, from birth to dying, has characteristic pain problems. Genetics, until recently, was rarely considered relevant to understanding pain, yet sophisticated laboratory studies and clinical observations have established genetic predispositions related to pain as an essential component of the field. The study of pain, therefore, now incorporates research in epidemiology and medical genetics as well as sociological and cultural studies.

The impact of the pain revolution is revealed by the contents of this textbook. The further we move from a stimulus-driven concept of pain, the better we recognize the validity of baffling pain syndromes that often have no obvious pathology to explain the presence of pain or its terrible intensity. Chronic pains become increasingly comprehensible when we extend our diagnostic search to consider multiple causal mechanisms.

We have a mission – all of us – to rectify the existing situation, for cancer pain as well as postsurgical pain, for pain in children and the elderly, and for any kind of severe pain which can be helped by sensible administration of drugs and other pain therapies. We must also teach patients to communicate better about their pain, and inform them that they have a right to freedom from pain, that each suffering human being deserves the best that the health professions have to offer. We must also get our message to those in government that pain is a major plague that saps the strength of society, that funds for research and therapy are urgently needed, and that regulations regarding the supply of drugs must be modified to reflect the needs of people in pain, not just the misdeeds of street addicts. If we can pursue these goals together – as scientists and therapists, as members of the full range of scientific and health professions – we can hope to meet the goal we all strive for: to help our fellow human beings who suffer pain.

Ronald Melzack
McGill University
Montreal, Quebec, Canada, 2006

Preface

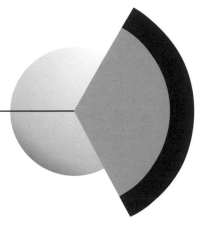

To suffer pain from time to time is part of the human condition. The treatment of people in pain is part of the daily life of many doctors, nurses and other professionals working in the health field. In October 2004, the slogan for a Global Day Against Pain promoted jointly by the International Association for the Study of Pain (IASP), the European Federation of IASP Chapters (EFIC) and the World Health Organization (WHO) was, 'The Treatment of Pain Should be a Human Right'. Despite this overwhelming evidence for the need for a sound knowledge of pain and its management to be a major focus for undergraduate and postgraduate education, this need is even yet not fully met.

During the past 40 years, knowledge of the biological, psychological and social aspects of pain has increased enormously. In developed countries, services for the treatment of pain have increased steadily. For example, most general hospitals have teams of doctors and nurses that deal with acute pain and especially postoperative pain. Major centres for population usually have one or more pain clinics for the treatment of difficult or more chronic pain problems and are staffed by teams, which, in their full form, involve doctors, psychologists, nurses, physiotherapists and possibly other health professionals. The hospice movement, now worldwide, was founded in London by Dame Cecily Saunders in the 1960s and has pioneered the treatment of pain and other symptoms of advanced malignant disease.

Education, involving understanding the nature of pain and its clinical presentation together with its management, must begin at an undergraduate level. In this way, a sound foundation for future learning is established and newly qualified health professionals will have a good working knowledge of pain analysis and treatment that they can apply with confidence to their patients.

This book has been written primarily for undergraduates in medicine, nursing and other professionals working in the field of medicine but, in addition, may be of interest to others including members of the lay public. The text is divided into three parts. The first part deals with the nature of pain and the complex changes that take place in the nervous system between an event causing damage to some part of the body and the experience of pain. That experience includes mental changes involving the emotions and cognitive functions, and it leads to changes in behaviour. We are able now to assess the severity of pain in various ways and an analysis of behaviour gives important clues to the source of pain, the ability of an individual to cope with pain and at times the possibility that acute pain will become chronic pain. The second part is devoted to a description of conditions that give rise to pain, both acute and chronic, and the relationship between pain and mental disorders. Emphasis is placed upon the importance of pain in the assessment of the patient's overall condition, and in order to make that as accurate as possible, a full pain history is required. A chapter is devoted to evaluation of the clinical history – a practical clinical skill that all clinicians should possess. The final part deals with the physical and psychological techniques used in the management of pain. Full coverage is given to the use of analgesics of various kinds and the main features of invasive techniques such as epidural anaesthesia, intradural drug delivery, nerve blocks, spinal cord stimulation and other methods including transcutaneous electrical stimulation of nerves, acupuncture and hypnosis. The role of pain management clinics is described. A chapter is devoted to cancer pain and another to the use of psychological techniques including cognitive/behavioural therapy, counselling, relaxation therapy and hypnosis.

Careful study of the contents of this book will both inform those who treat people in pain and, in turn, reduce the level of suffering from pain in the general population.

MRB, KHS, 2006

List of abbreviations

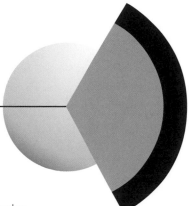

APS	acute pain service
APT	acute pain team
BMD	bone minimal density
COX	cyclo-oxygenase
CRPS	complex regional pain syndrome
CSF	cerebrospinal fluid
CT	computerized tomography
ECG	electrocardiograph
EFIC	European Federation of IASP Chapters
fMRI	functional magnetic resonance imaging
GABA	gamma amino butyric acid
GDP	gross domestic product
HADS	Hospital Anxiety and Depression Scale
5-HT	5-hydroxytryptamine
IASP	International Association for the Study of Pain
ITDD	intrathecal drug delivery
MEAC	minimum effective analgesic blood concentration
MLAC	minimum local anaesthetic concentration
MPQ	McGill Pain Questionnaire
MRI	magnetic resonance imaging
NHS	National Health Service
NMDA	N-methyl-D-aspartate
NNH	number needed to harm
NNT	number needed to treat
NSAID	non-steroidal anti-inflammatory drug
PCA	patient-controlled analgesia
PET	positron emission tomography
PHN	postherpetic neuralgia
PPI	Present Pain Index
PPT	Pain Perception Threshold

SCS	spinal cord stimulation
SF-MPQ	Short Form McGill Pain Questionnaire
SPT	Severe Pain Threshold
TENS	transcutaneous electrical nerve stimulation
VAS	Visual Analogue Scale
WHO	World Health Organization

The nature of pain

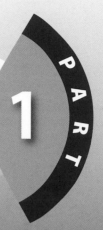

The nature of pain

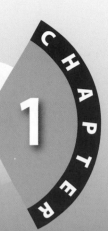

CHAPTER 1

Chapter objectives

After studying this chapter you should be able to:

1 Define the nature of pain.
2 Describe the historical developments of the concept of pain that lead ultimately to the definition of pain devised by the International Association for the Study of Pain.

Pain as a mental event

Pain is a psychological state, a mental experience and a product of consciousness. Although it is not experienced other than in the conscious state, reflex or stereotyped behaviours do occur when noxious stimuli are applied to an unconscious person.

Definition of pain

The accepted definition of pain, produced by the International Association for the Study of Pain, is as follows:

Pain is 'an unpleasant sensory and emotional experience associated with actual or potential damage, or described in terms of such damage, and pain is always subjective. Each individual learns the application of the word through experiences related to injury in early life'.

There are two important points that arise from this definition.

1 Pain is normally regarded as an indication that physical damage has occurred to, or is taking place within, the body. However, pain experience does not necessarily mean that damage has occurred and pain intensity may be far greater than the extent of an injury or a disease would suggest. Pain, therefore, is an inner experience generated within the brain by different combinations of physical and psychological factors. Its severity and the behaviour it evokes vary under the influence of external, social and cultural factors. Therefore, the same individual may respond differently to the same painful stimulus if their circumstances change.

2 Cognitive, emotional and behavioural components of pain are influenced by our past experience of pain and that of others in pain, in particular the members of our families. Therefore, individuals differ in their experience of pain and behave differently even when suffering similar common disorders (Box 1.1). Failure to recognize this simple fact often leads to poor management of pain because many clinicians have a fixed view of what people 'ought to feel' and how they 'should behave' when in pain.

Pain theories

Until the middle of the 20th century attempts to understand the nature of pain were divided between those who regarded pain

> **Box 1.1**
>
> ### The nature of pain
>
> - Pain is a mental experience.
> - It occurs only in the conscious state.
> - It is the result of sensory, emotional and cognitive activity in the brain influenced by past experiences from childhood onwards, family, social and cultural factors.
> - Pain is usually interpreted as being the result of tissue damage, although this is not necessarily the case.

primarily as a product of the mind and others who regarded it as due to physiological processes in the nervous system. The 'mind/body split' can be traced to the 17th century and did not begin to disappear until the middle of the 20th century.

The Specificity theory

This was first used to explain the nature of pain. To quote Ronald Melzack, a famous psychologist and neuroscientist: 'This theory states that a specific pain system carries messages directly from receptors in the skin to a pain centre in the brain'. It originated in a hypothesis proposed by Rene Descartes in the mid 17th century. He envisaged that the generation of pain resembled a man ringing a church bell – pulling one end of the bell rope results in a sound at the other. That process, when translated into human terms, means that stimulation of nerves in the skin results in the direct transfer of the sensation of pain from the skin to the brain (Fig. 1. 1). In the middle of the 19th century the discovery of the physical properties of the nervous system began to emerge and, with them, refinements in the theory. A growing awareness of anomalies in pain experience that could not be accounted for by the Specificity theory, however amended, resulted ultimately in its abandonment.

With increasing knowledge of the nervous system, refinement of the Specificity theory led to the belief by physiologists that sensations are a consequence of stimulating specific sensory nerves that differ in their intrinsic properties. Only in this way could one account for the differences in sensation resulting from stimulation of the skin by touch, heat and cold. In 1842 Johannes Muller said that differences in sensation were due to differences in specific energies in nerves, or to special properties of different areas of the brain. He did not question the underlying assumption that information travelled directly from the source of stimulation to the brain. Max von Frey, in

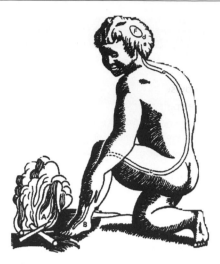

Fig 1.1 Descartes' model of pain. Descartes' concept of the pain pathway (1644): 'If for example fire (A) comes near the foot (B), the minute the particles of this fire, which as you know move with great velocity, have the power to set in motion the spot of the skin of the foot they touch, and by means pullling on the delicate thread (cc) which is attached to the spot on the skin, they open up at the same instant the pore (de) against which the delicate thread ends, just as by pulling at one end of a rope one makes to strike at the same instant a bell which hangs at the other'.
Reproduced with permission from Melzack R The puzzle of pain: Penguin Science of Behaviour. Penguin Books 1973.

the 1880s, next proposed that each mode of sensation must have its own conduction system to the brain. He defined four sensations in the skin: touch, warmth, cold and pain. Microscopic and physiological experiments revealed structures in the skin thought to give rise to three of the four sensations, the exception being pain. Specific sensory end organs, or terminals, were named after their discoverers and included the Meissner corpuscles (touch), the Ruffini end organs (warmth) and the Krause end bulbs (cold). Specific sensory terminals could not be found for pain and therefore free nerve endings found in the skin and around the hair follicles were described by von Frey as pain receptors. Later histological and physiological work failed to link the receptors with specific sensations, but free nerve endings were found to have specific properties that led to the development of the different sensations. Von Frey did link specific sensations to receptors in the skin and others later traced their neural connections into the central nervous system and described the way in which they result in different sensations.

Pattern theory

In 1894 Goldsheider proposed that, to evoke a sensation, a stimulus should exceed a threshold in order to generate neural activity. Also, the processes of convergence and summation of impulses from peripheral nerves reaching the dorsal horns of the spinal cord seemed important in pain generation. Pain could occur, therefore, either when the thresholds for stimulation for normally non-noxious stimuli, such as touch or heat, were exceeded or when, as a result of pathological processes, the summation of impulses was increased to the point where a normally non-noxious stimulus became painful; this experience is known as 'allodynia'.

In certain pathological states, there is an unusually long period between stimulation of the skin and the experience of pain, for example in tabes dorsalis (a condition due to syphilis that was common in Goldsheider's day), which suggested that there must be pathways consisting of multisynaptic nerves and, therefore, a more slowly conducting system conveying information to the brain. Tactile sensations were felt much sooner than pain; therefore it was believed that neural activity for touch must travel more quickly and more directly through the dorsal columns of the spinal cord to the brain.

Goldsheider introduced the concept of specific patterning of nerve impulses as a prerequisite for pain experience and alterations in pattern formation as a necessary preliminary for abnormal pain states.

In the 1940s and 1950s, experimental work revealed that a one-to-one relationship existed between peripheral nerve fibre size and the quality of sensory experience generated, but the belief in a direct pathway from the periphery to the brain persisted. On the basis of animal experiments, Keele suggested in 1957 that the anterolateral quadrant of the spinal cord was the site of major pain pathways. Confirmation occurred later with the abolition of chronic pain in humans when nerve fibres in the anterolateral tracts were divided in a surgical procedure known as cordotomy.

Like Goldsheider, Livingstone (1943) stated that abnormal patterns of nerve impulses from peripheral nerves in the conditions of phantom limb, causalgia and neuralgias initiate abnormal patterns of nerve activity in the spinal cord. This was the result of summation that gave rise to activity in the brain where pain is generated. He went further and said that, in order to explain those abnormalities of neuronal activity within the spinal cord, nerve impulses must spread to nearby nerve cells initiating reverberating circuits. As a result, non-noxious stimuli could give rise to abnormal pain sensations. Also, associated autonomic and muscular activity such as sweating and jerking of the limbs was said to generate further abnormal impulse activity. It was Livingstone's view, therefore, that abnormal activity in the spinal cord, once generated, could become self-sustaining through reverberating circuits in groups of neurons in the cord. A mechanism of this type has been demonstrated recently. Livingstone said that attempts to control pain by cutting peripheral nerves would fail because of the presence of the abnormal mechanism in the spinal cord, and this observation is in keeping with clinical experience. He stated that modification or abolition of sensation from abnormal nerves by injections of local anaesthetic could lead to reversal of the processes in the cord. Recently, anaesthetists have attempted to prevent the development of phantom limb pain using regional anaesthesia techniques immediately before and after surgery, but to date the results have been mixed and inconclusive. Furthermore, work on the spinal cord has revealed that cutting nerve pathways within the anterolateral columns (cordotomy) does not usually reduce or abolish pain caused by abnormal nerve activity more peripherally for more than a few months only in most cases. Therefore, other pathways for conduction must exist and if summation of nerve impulses does take place in the spinal cord then there is a process that, under normal circumstances, inhibits it. Loss or destruction of that mechanism would itself lead to abnormal pain states. The mechanism proposed was one in which a rapidly conducting nerve fibre system would inhibit a more slowly conducting system responsible for pain generation. With loss of dominance of the fast conducting system, burning pain and hyperalgesia (increased sensitivity to painful stimuli) would develop. Nordenbos (1959) stated that small diameter nerve fibres in peripheral nerves conduct impulses for pain generation and that larger diameter fibre activity inhibits transmission of the small fibres. In addition, he said that a multisynaptic ascending conduction system in the spinal cord would explain the failure of cordotomy to abolish pain permanently, because through this system nerve impulses could 'leak' to higher centres. He did not demonstrate his hypothesis by experimentation, but the concept was a major advance and undermined further the specificity theory. Nordenbos prepared the way for the development of the 'Gate Theory' proposed by Melzack & Wall in 1965 (Figs 1.2 and 1. 3). It formed the foundation for much of the future basic research in pain science and, in particular, the understanding of spinal cord mechanisms control-

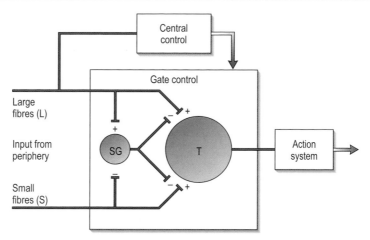

Fig 1.2 Gate control theory I (GCT-I). L, the large diameter fibres. S, the small diameter fibres. The fibres project to the substantia gelatinosa (SG) and the first central transmission (T) cells. The inhibitory effect exerted by the SG on the afferent fibre terminals is increased by activity in L fibres and decreased by activity in S fibres. The central control trigger is represented by a line running from the large fibre system to the central control mechanisms; these mechanisms, in turn, project back to the gate control system. The T cells project to the action system. (+, excitation; −, inhibition.) Reprinted with permission from Melzack & Wall 1965, p. 975. Pain mechanisms: a new theory. Science 150:971–979. Copyright 1965 AAAS.

ling pain generation and modulation in the spinal cord (Box 1.2).

Psychological theories of pain

The origins of psychological theories of pain are attributable to Aristotle, who defined five senses – sight, hearing, smell, taste and touch, but set pain apart and described it as a 'passion of the soul' – a state of feeling. His views persisted for a thousand years and other famous physicians, including Avicenna in the 11th century and Spinoza in the 17th century, also regarded pain as an emotion. Thomas Sydenham, perhaps the most famous physician in the 17th century and known as 'The English Hippocrates', had the belief that the condition of hysteria, the most common of all chronic diseases in his time, was primarily psychological in origin and that pain was one of its possible features. The physician Benjamin Brodie, said in 1837 that certain forms of pain were not attributable to physical conditions but to hysteria and he claimed that in upper class women four-fifths of joint pains were hysterical in origin! He stated that a number of psychological factors, including fear

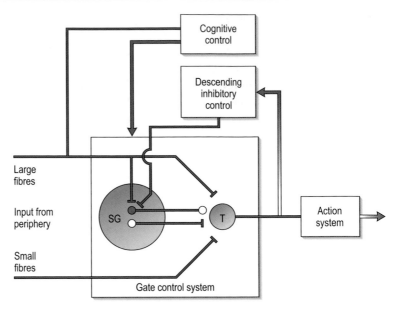

Fig 1.3 Gate control theory II. A later model which includes excitatory (white circle) and inhibitor (black circle) links from the substantia gelatinosa (SG) to the transmission (T) cells as well as descending inhibitory control from the brainstem systems. The round knob at the end of the inhibitory link implies that its actions may be presynaptic, postsynaptic, or both. All connections are excitatory, except the inhibitory link from SG to T cell. Reproduced from Melzack & Wall 1983, The challenge of pain, Basic Books, New York.

Box 1.2

The history of physiologically based pain theories

- From the mid 17th to the 20th century it was believed that pain arose as a result of stimulation of the skin with direct transfer of sensation to the brain, (the Specificity theory).

- Discovery of the electrical properties of nerves in the 19th century resulted in the view that specific nerves for pain and other sensations existed.

- A number of specific nerve endings in the skin were identified as the origin of the sensations of touch, heat and cold and free nerve endings were thought to be where pain originated. Evidence for specific 'end organs' was later discounted.

- In 1965 the Gate Theory of Pain established the basic pattern of neuronal activity in the peripheral nerves, spinal cord and brain, for the generation and modulation of pain.

and suggestion, were factors in the causation of hysteria. The definition of the term 'hysteria' in the 18th and 19th centuries was quite different from definitions found in textbooks of mental illness at the present time. The important point, however, is that Sydenham and others recognised that pain could be generated or altered by psychological as well as physical causes. Freud, early in the 20th century, proposed that pain could be generated by the mind – a concept that is in accordance with our current belief that the experience of pain may occur in the absence of noxious peripheral stimulation and in certain emotional states (e.g. depression and anxiety). He emphasized an association between pain and the mental processes, of repression, of aggression and of guilt and he therefore proposed that pain could act as a punishment of the self. It could be seen also as a means of communicating emotions of various kinds to others at the unconscious level and, in particular, anger and a need for help. Clinicians of today recognize that pain may have these functions at times without the sufferer being aware that pain is not necessarily an indicator of tissue damage. Not all doctors accepted this relationship until recently, but regarded pain that had an obvious physical cause as 'organic' and pain that did not as 'neurotic' or even imaginary.

Thomas Szasz re-emphasized in the 1950s that, apart from its value as an indicator of physical injury and disease, pain could become an unconscious form of aggression towards others, and that suffering pain could relieve guilt. George Engel went further and suggested that in the general population there are individuals who have 'a pain-prone personality'. They had, he said, a family history of painful conditions, came from lower socioeconomic groups, had undergone frequent surgical operations and were poorly adjusted sexually. 'Pain-prone' patients were said to exhibit self-punitive behaviour and to experience pain at times when they could have experienced pleasure, in other words when life's problems were minimal. Such individuals, when exposed to pain, were said to be unusually tolerant of it. Research into the various aspects of the pain-prone personality have not confirmed that it exists, but there is evidence that psychological trauma in early life is associated with a greater likelihood of developing chronic pain in adult life. For example, physical and sexual abuse in childhood are recognised as predisposing factors to, and enhancers of, chronic pain that does not have an obvious physical cause.

Physiological considerations dominated scientific and medical thought during the greater part of the 19th century and psychological aspects of pain were relatively neglected. Laymen and doctors alike regarded pain as either 'real', meaning that it had a physical origin, or 'imaginary', which carried the belief with it that pain was a product of the mind and therefore not real. The perception by pain sufferers that others regard their pain as 'imaginary' creates great distress and a feeling of disregard for their suffering. This illustrates very clearly how the mind/body split, originating with Descartes, operated and how frequently this disadvantaged the sufferer. Patients with chronic pain may say even now in an accusing voice 'so you think it's all in my mind doctor' when they are firmly convinced that their pain has a physical basis because they too share the belief that pain always indicates a physical abnormality, a disease, or an injury. There is ample evidence available that pain may be experienced in the absence of disease or injury and that complaints of pain may be out of proportion to any physical abnormality detected. Pain plays a significant role in interpersonal behaviour. It can also be used as a means of expressing a variety of emotions or controlling the behaviour of others, or both. Such behaviour is not consciously determined, except when the individual is malingering, using the symptom to gain access to powerful drugs, or perhaps to obtain compensation for injury.

Box 1.3

Psychological theories of pain

- From the time of Aristotle until the 19th century, pain was regarded as an emotion. In the 17th century, ideas put forward by Descartes resulted in the separation of the functions of mind and body up to the early 20th century. As a result, pain was regarded as either physical in origin or as imaginary, or neurotic, if an obvious physical cause for it could not be found.

- Freud linked pain to unconscious mental conflicts. The psychosomatic school of the early 20th century linked unconscious psychic conflicts and personality attributes with specific diseases, several of which are painful. These theories have not proved to be sound scientifically.

- Modern approaches to the role of psychological mechanisms in pain generation and modulation, and to associated behaviour patterns, are based upon Behavioural Theory and Cognitive Theory.

The psychological theories of Freud and the psychosomatic school applied to pain have not, for the most part, proved to be valid when submitted to scientific scrutiny. A significant psychological breakthrough came, however, in the period 1970–1990 when the Behavioural Theory and Cognitive Theories, both soundly based scientifically, proved to have a powerful role in the understanding of pain at a psychological level and were useful as tools in pain management (Box 1.3). Their appearance revolutionized attitudes to pain management and they are described in detail in Chapter 5.

Self-assessment questions

Answer 'True' or 'False' to the following statements:

1.1 Pain is:

   a. An indicator of physical damage to the body
   b. A mental experience with sensory, emotional and cognitive elements arising from damage to the body
   c. A set of complex behaviours reflecting damage to the body
   d. A mental experience with sensory, cognitive and emotional elements that does not always signify bodily damage
   e. The antithesis of pleasure

Pain in society

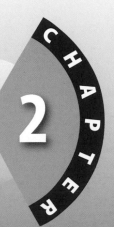

Chapter objectives

After studying this chapter you should be able to:

1 Understand why it is difficult to assess the extent to which pain is present in the general population.

2 Use information taken from epidemiological studies conducted on the specific conditions of migraine and back pain to illustrate the extent of pain due to these causes.

3 Give an account of the cost of back pain in social and economic terms and to illustrate the need to balance economic cost against risks to health when using analgesic drugs and other pain management techniques.

The social burden of pain

Pain is a major health problem, but what is its scale, how many people suffer from pain, what proportion receives adequate treatment, what are the success rates of different treatments and what is the cost of pain and its management to society? Answers to these questions are needed to make adequate provision for both the prevention and the treatment of pain, and these issues are the legitimate concern of epidemiological surveys. There are, however, significant barriers to population studies in the field of pain because it is present in different forms in a wide range of disorders. Although pain is a symptom of many diseases it might be regarded as the primary disorder in conditions such as migraine, trigeminal neuralgia and other forms of nerve damage, and in chronic pain states where pain is the overwhelming predominating symptom. The International Association for the Study of Pain, a body concerned with pain research and clinical management of pain, has classified pain syndromes; at the latest count there were 600. For example, 36 were generalized syndromes, and 60 affected the head and neck, 35 the upper limbs, 154 the thoracic and cervical spine regions, 136 the lumbar, sacral, coccygeal, spinal and nerve root regions, 85 the trunk and 18 the lower limbs. As each syndrome has its own epidemiological profile, the problems for those conducting epidemiological studies in this area of medicine are formidable.

Having defined a pain syndrome the next problem is to define the duration of pain. The International Association for the Study of Pain devised three categories; acute pain (lasting less than 1 month), subacute pain (lasting 1 to 6 months) and chronic pain (lasting 6 months or more), but not all published epidemiological studies use this form of classification.

The epidemiology of pain

Before describing the contribution of different epidemiological studies to our understanding of the issues outlined in the first paragraph of this chapter, it is necessary to understand the meaning of the terms used to describe the extent that problems, for example pain, occur in populations. Box 2.1 defines the key terms, prevalence and incidence, used in this chapter.

Prevalence studies of pain in hospital reveal a higher level of moderate to severe pain than in the community. Studies of acute postoperative pain show that it remains poorly managed

Box 2.1

Definitions of epidemiological terms

- **Prevalence:** The percentage of individuals in a known population who have the symptoms being studied at some point during a specific time, i.e. 1 month prevalence, 1 year prevalence.

- **Point prevalence:** The percentage of individuals in a known population with the symptoms on the day of interview.

- **Lifetime prevalence:** The percentage of individuals in a known population who have had the symptom at some time in their lives.

- **Incidence:** The percentage of people in a known population who develop symptoms during a specified period of time, i.e. report injuries or pain within a specific period.

despite the establishment of acute pain services in many hospitals. In 1990 a landmark report from the joint British Royal Colleges of Surgeons and Anaesthetists concerning pain after surgery recommended that acute pain services be established in acute hospitals. An audit commission report in 1997 showed that between 10 and 20% of those who returned home on the day of surgery experienced unacceptable levels of pain immediately afterwards. Uncontrolled pain was the reason that many day-surgery patients had to stay in hospital overnight rather than go home as planned; this has social and economic implications. A study in 2001 reported that over three-quarters of patients having elective abdominal or orthopaedic surgery had moderate or severe postoperative pain. A review of acute pain services in 2004 showed that national coverage by acute pain services in the UK is far from being achieved; this is largely because of organizational and political barriers. Studies show that patients have different relative preferences for the trade-off between good analgesia and side effects. Healthcare professionals need to understand these to best meet the patients' expectations and needs.

A review of recent epidemiological studies of pain in the adult general population revealed that chronic pain, present for more than 6 months, occurs in between 45 and 65% of the population with musculoskeletal pains. Follow-up surveys show that chronic pain often persists for many years. A large European telephone survey of over 13 000 people showed that moderate or severe pain was a problem for 18% of those

Box 2.2

The personal consequences of chronic pain – a European study

- 50–65% less able or unable to exercise, enjoy normal sleep, perform household duties, attend social activities, drive a car, or have sexual relations.

- 25% relationships with family and friends strained or broken.

- 33% less able or unable to maintain an independent life.

- 20% depressed because of pain.

- 17% suffered so badly that some days they wanted to die.

- 39% felt that their pain was inadequately managed. In such cases their doctor did not view their pain as a problem.

From the European Journal of Pain (in press), Brevik H, Ventafridda V, Collett B. The pain in Europe survey: detailed results and analysis. Copyright 2005, with permission from the European Federation of Chapters of the International Association of the Study of Pain.

surveyed; there was wide variation between countries ranging from 11 to 27%. Degenerative conditions and back pain were the commonest problems. Severe pain was experienced by about a third of 2400 people assessed in more detail and it was slightly more common in women than in men. In a third of people, pain was present every day. Pain resulted in loss of time from work and social activities in many chronic pain sufferers. A fifth of those surveyed had been diagnosed as being depressed because of pain (Box 2.2).

Many studies show that patients with cancer-related pain often have inadequate pain management in hospital. Approximately 30–40% of patients with cancer on active therapy report pain, and this rises to 70–90% of patients with advanced disease. About 76% of patients with chronic lung disease report pain during the final year of life, with more than half rating pain as 'very distressing'. Similarly 32% of patients with end-stage heart failure and 65% of stroke patients experience pain in their last year of life.

Less is known about the prevalence of pain in children than in adults and methods of pain assessment in younger children and neonates are under development. Some studies in neonates have suggested that early pain experiences can have an effect on pain perception and painful conditions in adult life. One study revealed that, of 6000 children at home, 54% had experienced pain within the previous 3 months, and a quarter of those had had repeated or chronic pain. Pain was most common in the limbs, head and abdomen, and half the children had more than one type of pain. Girls over 12 years of age recorded more chronic pain and multiple pains than boys or younger girls. Services for children with chronic pain are poorly established in most countries.

Specific epidemiological studies

Epidemiological studies of two common conditions, namely headache and back pain, illustrate some of the basic principles of epidemiology and the uses of epidemiological data in pain research.

Migraine headache

The first step in any epidemiological study is to define the condition in terms that are agreed as widely as possible. For example, in 2004 The International Headache Society produced agreed new definitions including migraine with and without an aura and episodic tension-type headache (Boxes 2.3 and 2.4).

Box 2.3

Forms of migraine

1 Migraine without aura

2 Migraine with aura:
   a. Typical aura with a migraine headache
   b. Typical aura with non-migraine headache
   c. Typical aura without headache
   d. Familial hemiplegic migraine
   e. Sporadic hemiplegic migraine
   f. Basilar type migraine

3 Childhood periodic syndromes that are common antecedents of migraine:
   a. Cyclical vomiting
   b. Abdominal migraine
   c Benign paroxysmal vertigo of childhood

Other migrainous disorders

International Headache Society 2004. From: The International Classification of Headache Disorders, 2edn. Cephalalgia, vol. 24, suppl 1, 2004. Reproduced with permission of Blackwell Publishing, Oxford.

Box 2.4

Forms of tension-type headache

1 Infrequent episodic tension-type headache.
   (<12 attacks per year).

2 Frequent episodic tension-type headache.
   (>1 day per month but <15 days per month)

3 Chronic tension-type headache
   (15 days per month or more for at least 3 months).

All types of headache may or may not be associated with pericranial tenderness.

International Headache Society 2004. From: The International Classification of Headache Disorders, 2edn. Cephalalgia, vol. 24, suppl 1, 2004. Reproduced with permission of Blackwell Publishing, Oxford.

Table 2.1 Lifetime prevalence of common primary and secondary headaches in percentages and with 95% confidence limits

Headaches	% Lifetime prevalence (both sexes) and range
Primary	
Migraine without aura	9 (7–11)
Migraine with aura	6 (5–8)
Episodic tension-type headache	66 (62–69)
Chronic tension-type headache	3 (2–5)
Cluster headache	0.1 (0–1)
Secondary	
Associated with head trauma	4 (2–5)
Vascular disorders	1 (0–2)
Non-vascular intracranial disorders	0.5 (0–1)
Hangover	72 (68–75)
Fever headache	63 (59–66)

Adapted from Rasmussen BK, Olesen J 1992 Symptomatic and non-symptomatic headaches in a general population. Neurology 42: 1225–1231. Reproduced with permission from Lippincott, Williams & Wilkins.

On the basis of original criteria of 1992, the lifetime prevalence of migraine and secondary headaches was calculated (Table 2.1). The 1 year prevalence overall was 10–20% (6% for men and 15–18% for women). These data reveal that the ratio of male to female sufferers is 1 to 2 or 3. Contrasting migraine with an aura (often termed classical migraine) and without aura (often known as common migraine) shows that the former is commoner in women. They have migraine with an aura more frequently than migraine without one. Amongst men there is an even division between those who have migraine with and without an aura. Prevalence studies give a clue to the possible reason for the male to female differences because they do not emerge until children are about 11 years old at a time when rapid hormonal changes begin to occur. This and other factors have led to the belief that female hormones are linked to the greater extent to which women suffer from migraine, and migraine with an aura.

Migraine surveys reveal that the common age of onset is in the second and third decades of life and after the fourth decade its prevalence falls.

For many years it was believed that migraine is a condition that afflicts the more intelligent and affluent members of society, but studies of the relevant demographic and social factors have shown that this is not the case. However, it is probable that in countries where healthcare is a direct cost to the individual the more affluent seek medical advice more often. Therefore, epidemiological surveys need to take account of both socioeconomic status and health-related behaviours.

Studies of tension-type headaches have revealed that about 60% of sufferers experience them about 1 day per month or less, 40% experience them several times a month, but less than 5% experience headache more than 180 days in the year. The Danish study, from which these figures were taken, showed that just over 40% of the population with tension-type head-ache were not prevented from carrying out daily activities, whereas just less than 60% of the same group were restricted to a moderate or even a severe degree. The lifetime preva-lences of tension and other forms of headache are given in Tables 2.1 and 2.2.

Tension-type headache occurs fairly uniformly across all social and economic groups.

Low back pain

It has been estimated that the lifetime prevalence of low back pain is in the order of 50 to 84%. The wide range expressed by these figures reflects the different criteria used in different studies and variations in the ages of the populations studied. Despite the extensive nature of low back pain, degenerative changes and radiological findings in the lumbar spine are poor predictors of episodes of low back pain. A clear physical cause

Table 2.2 Lifetime prevalence of common non-primary or secondary headaches in percentages and with 95% confidence limits

Headaches associated with	% Lifetime prevalence (both sexes) and range
Metabolic disorders	22 (19–25)
Disorders of nose or sinuses	15 (12–17)
Disorders of the eyes	3 (2–4)
Disorders of the neck	1 (0–2)
Disorders of the ears	0.5 (0–1)
Cranial neuralgias	0.5 (0–1)

Adapted from Rasmussen BK, Olesen J 1992 Symptomatic and non-symptomatic headaches in a general population. Neurology 42: 1225–1231. Reproduced with permission from Lippincott, Williams & Wilkins.

for an episode of back pain is found in only a small proportion of sufferers. In contrast to lifetime prevalence, figures for 1 month prevalence range between 19 and 43%, and for annual prevalence they range between 40 and 50%. However, despite this high prevalence, fewer than 10% of episodes of low back pain result in consultations by individuals with their family doctors. In fact, it is often stated that 50% of those with simple back pain will have improved within a week and 90% within a month. However, this still means that significant numbers of individuals experience pain that persists and for which they seek help. Even amongst those who do not consult their general practitioner it is known that a proportion may not have completely recovered from their pain 12 months later. Therefore prevalence rates for consultations with family doctors do not reflect the true extent of low back pain in the general population.

The prevalence of low back pain is said to rise with age and that the rise continues up to the age of 50 to 60 years, being greater in men than in women. Those figures are clearly a simplification because they do not take account of occupation and ethnic mix.

As a cause of ill health in a Swedish study conducted in 1996, 3–5% of individuals aged 16 to 44 years, 11–12% of those aged 45 to 64 and 9–11% of those aged 65 to 84 had low back pain. It is the most common cause of chronic sickness in men

Table 2.3 Low back pain and disability rates by country

Country	Population (millions)	Sick days (millions per year)	Percentage of work force	Days absent (per patient per year)	Level of insurance benefit (%)
United States	240	20	2	9	0–80
Canada	23	10	2	20	40–90
Great Britain	55	33	2	30	0–80
West Germany	61	16	4	10	100 (0–4 wks)
					80 (5–8 wks)
					60 (9 wks)
The Netherlands	14	4	4	25	80
Sweden 1980	8	7	3	25	90
1983	8	13	5	30	90
1987	8.5	28	8	40	100

From Fordyce WE 1995 Back pain in the workplace. Management of disability in non-specific conditions.
Reproduced with permission from the International Association for the Study of Pain (IASP Press) Seattle.

and women less than 64 years of age, and the second most common in those over 65, when circulatory problems dominate.

Epidemiological studies with regard to the nature of low back pain concludes that it should not be regarded as acute, recurrent or chronic, but as a recurrent intermittent and episodic problem. Therefore, when assessing a patient the lifelong pattern of back pain (e.g. total number of days in pain per year) is a satisfactory predictor of future episodes.

Table 2.3 illustrates the situation in six countries. In terms of days absent from work in large populations the problem appears to be greater in Canada, Great Britain, the Netherlands and Sweden, when compared with the United States and Germany. The consequences of low back pain in terms of 'sick days' (days absent from work), the percentage of the work force involved and the levels of insurance benefit paid shows that the data relate to low back pain in working people rather than the community at large. The table reveals the potential economic consequences of low back pain and a major use of epidemiological studies in the examination of economic burdens of a physical disorder to society. Table 2.4 gives a more detailed

Table 2.4 Consequences of the back pain epidemic in the United Kingdom

Sickness absence	52.6 million certified working days 1988–99 (largest single cause; 12.5% of total sick days)
Lost output	Estimated loss (1987–98) £2 billion
General practitioner consults	Estimated 2 million annually
Hospital outpatient consults	Estimated 300 000 annually
Hospital inpatient episodes	Estimated 100 000 (1989–90)
Severe disability	50–1000 people severely affected in an average health district of 250 000 population

From Frank A 1993 Regular review: low back pain. BMJ 306: 901–909. Reproduced with permission from the BMJ Publishing Group.

picture of the actual consequences of back pain in the work force and upon the economy of Great Britain in 1993.

The examples chosen to illustrate the use of epidemiological techniques in the study of pain do not deal with the causes of the conditions concerned, the risk factors for their development, the question of the relative contributions of physical, psychological and social factors, or methods of management and outcome criteria. These will be dealt with when the clinical features of headache, back pain and other pain disorders are considered further in Chapters 7 and 8.

The economics of pain

Pain has an economic cost to the individual (loss of earnings, normal daily activities, socialization and leisure time), to society (production losses, invalidity benefits), and the health provider (costs of outpatient and inpatient attendances, drugs, anaesthetics, other treatments and investigations) (Box 2.5). The costs to society have been calculated in various ways as shown in the following examples. The cost to employers of the common condition of migraine has been calculated at £60–£70 million per year in the United Kingdom. In 1998 the direct cost of back pain was said to be £1 632 million, of which about one-third was related to costs in the private healthcare sector. It was estimated, however, that the costs of informal care and

> **Box 2.5**
>
> ## The economic and social costs of pain
>
> - Impaired health and associated disability has economic costs to sufferers, their carers, and society.
> - Costs to the individual are measurable in terms of lost income and reduction in activities of daily life, including ability to work, be domestically and socially active and follow leisure interests.
> - Cost to society include lost working days and production, direct medical costs related to investigation and treatment, and social benefits for the sick and disabled.
> - The cost of drugs to the NHS is very high. These costs should be borne in mind by prescribers who must also balance the cost of drugs against both their efficacy and their safety.

lost production were actually about ten times greater (£10 668 million). These figures indicate that the cost of back pain healthcare in the United Kingdom is of the order of 1.5% of the gross domestic product (GDP) and close to the figure of 1.7% calculated for the Netherlands in 1991. Back pain, therefore, is one of the costliest conditions for which an economic analysis has been carried out. It imposes a greater economic burden than coronary heart disease, Alzheimer's disease, stroke, insulin dependent diabetes, epilepsy, depression and several other major medical conditions.

In Wales in 2000, £31 million was spent on analgesics and, of that, £17 million was spent on non-steroidal anti-inflammatory drugs (NSAIDs). The role of these drugs in pain management is discussed in Chapters 15 to 17. When considering the costs of pain management with this class of drugs, it should be noted that the first identified (cyclo-oxygenase-1 or COX-1 inhibitors) may result in bleeding from the upper gastrointestinal tract or abnormalities of blood coagulation, especially amongst the elderly. These side effects are significantly less when certain COXIBs (COX-2) drugs are used the latter may have significant adverse cardiovascular effects. There is therefore a need to balance the therapeutic effect and costs of a drug against its dangers (costs in health terms to the patient and in cash terms to society).

Clearly the costs of pain management are complex and go well beyond the issue of the costs of diagnosis and treatment to the National Health Service (NHS) and include those to society and to the individual and carers.

Self-assessment questions

2.1 Define the term 'prevalence' – how does it differ from the term incidence?

2.2 Which of the following are *not* included in the definition of 'common migraine'?
a. Pulsating headache
b. Nausea and/or vomiting
c. Visual scotoma
d. Tight/pressing pain

2.3 The lifetime prevalence of low back pain is in the order of:
a. 19–43%
b. 15–30%
c. 50–80%

2.4 What proportion of individuals who develop low back pain recover within:
a. A week
b. A month?

2.5 List the economic and social costs of pain.

The measurement of pain

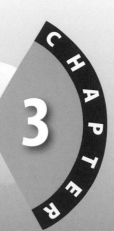

CHAPTER

3

Chapter objectives

After studying this chapter you should be able to:

1 Describe the different methods used to measure pain in human experiments and clinical practice and to assess their strengths and weaknesses.

2 Give reasons for the use of one or other of the methods in research and clinical situations taking account of the age, cultural background, cognitive function and language of the subjects.

3 Devise a pain assessment schedule for individuals with acute or chronic pain.

4 Understand that sex and gender influence pain.

5 Understand that race and ethnicity alter pain perception.

6 Appreciate that pain in neonates and children and the elderly may have different characteristics.

Pain assessment in man

Measurements of pain are used clinically to assess pain and its treatment, and in the laboratory to assess pain in experiments on man and animals. They are used to learn more about the effectiveness of methods of pain control, including the value of analgesic drugs for acute and chronic pain and the use of psychological techniques, especially in the management of chronic pain states (Box 3.1). Methods of pain assessment in animals will not be addressed.

Pain is a subjective experience, but the physiological changes that accompany it may be measured. These may include changes in heart rate, muscle tension, skin conductance and electrical activity in the brain; these changes are most consistent in acute rather than chronic pain. The physiological

Box 3.1

Measurement of pain

- Pain thresholds are measured using stimulus-dependent methods. Two thresholds may be identified – the Pain Perception Threshold (PPT) and the Severe Pain Threshold (SPT). The interval between the thresholds is a measure of pain tolerance.

- The PPT varies little between people in normal circumstances, but is lowered by damage to the peripheral nerves, for example in neuropathic states. The SPT and therefore, level of tolerance, varies widely within and between individuals as a result of personal, environmental and cultural influences. The SPT and level of tolerance are raised by pain-relieving techniques.

- The most commonly used clinical measurements of pain are response dependent and include the VAS, word scales of varying complexity, e.g. the McGill Pain Questionnaire, and non-verbal scales, e.g. the Faces Rating Scale used with children.

- The location and nature of pain may be recorded using a pain diagram.

- The use of a pain diary allows patients to record pain, activity and analgesic use when they are in their domestic and work environment.

- Pain is assessed by observation of pain-related behaviours, many of which are characteristic for acute and chronic pain disorders. Discrepancies between behaviours representing disability and reported levels of pain are clinically significant.

measures described are used chiefly in laboratory studies when observing human and animal subjects whereas, in contrast, self-report measures are favoured in clinical practice.

The dimensions of pain

Pain sensation may be experienced as aching, burning, cutting, stabbing, or other sensations. These qualities may change in their nature and pattern and this, together with their anatomical location, is often of diagnostic value. We have the ability to locate the site of noxious stimulation. This varies considerably, for example location of the pain of an injury to the surface of the body is accurate, although this may vary to some extent depending upon the local density of sensory neurons. In contrast, pain of visceral origin is often poorly located. In several conditions it manifests its presence by referral to sites on the body surface that can be distant from the affected organ. This occurs with inflammation of the gallbladder when pain is referred to the tip of the right shoulder, and in myocardial infarction when pain is felt in the chest, left arm and, at times, the left side of the jaw.

Afferent impulses generated by noxious stimulation are received by the sensory cortex and, at the same time, lead to cognitive activity. The individual appraises the significance of pain against a background of earlier memories and experiences, and together with the emotions generated, this changes perception of the significance of pain. As a result a range of characteristic behaviours develops. Acute pain gives rise to rapid withdrawal from the cause of pain, together with a drive to seek relief by one means or another, whereas chronic pain results in a variety of complex behavioural activities. These occur as the person adjusts to a greater or lesser extent to the presence of pain and its significance. The coping strategies adopted by a person and their family are often very important in those with chronic pain.

Pain thresholds

A number of methods have been devised for measuring pain. The application of any form of sensory stimulus, for example mechanical, thermal or electrical, will if increased steadily, change in quality until a point is reached at which pain is experienced. This is the lower of two pain thresholds – the Pain Perception Threshold (PPT). If the strength of the stimulus is

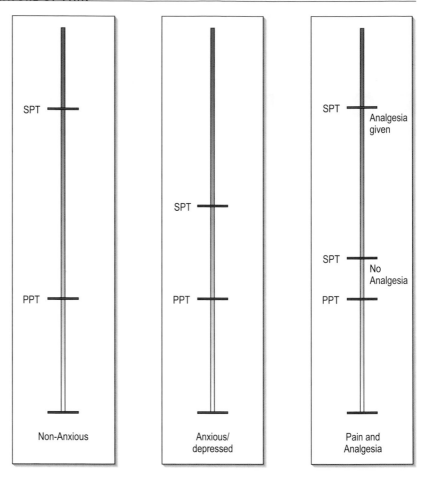

Fig 3.1 The effects of anxiety/depression and analgesia on pain thresholds for mechanical and thermal noxious stimuli (SPT = Severe Pain Threshold; PPT = Pain Perception Threshold).

increased, a second point is reached where the pain experienced becomes unbearable and this is the Severe Pain Threshold (SPT). The interval between the two thresholds is a measure of an individual's tolerance of stimulus-induced pain (Fig. 3.1). The process described involves the detection of physiologically determined thresholds using specific stimuli. This contrasts with measures used widely by clinicians in which patients evaluate pain on a psychological scale of pain magnitudes, for example using the Visual Analogue Scale (VAS) or simple word-based category scales described later in this chapter.

There is little variation in the lower of the two thresholds described between the sexes and different social and ethnic groups, but it is lowered in neuropathic pain disorders where there is damage to peripheral nerves. Values for the SPT vary widely both within and between individuals depending upon the circumstances in which pain occurs, the significance of the pain to the individual, and ethnic and cultural factors. There is evidence too that personality characteristics influence the level of pain tolerance. In general, pain tolerance is lower in women than in men and in more emotional people, for example those who are experiencing anxiety or depression, or both. Thresholds appear to be lower in clerical workers than in manual workers who have jobs in which minor or major injuries are common. Both thresholds, and especially the SPT, and therefore tolerance, are raised by the pharmacological effects of analgesic drugs, and by the reduction of anxiety. In about 30% of the population placebos, which are pharmacologically inert preparations, increase the SPT and therefore tolerance for pain – at least in the short term.

Self-report and observational measures

The Visual Analogue Scale

In the mid 1960s the Visual Analogue Scale (VAS), which was originally used to measure mood intensity (e.g. anxiety), was introduced to record the intensity of severity of pain experiences. It is very simple and ratings lie between two possible extremes, which are, 'I do not have any pain' and 'my pain could not be worse'. By using a scale of 0 to 100, or 0 to 10, quantification of the severity of pain is obtained (Fig. 3.2). This is done by asking patients to assess their pain at specific times and to mark the 10 centimetre line at a point that reflects their pain. The mark should refer to the pain being experienced currently and not to pain felt at some time previously because our ability to remember the intensity of previous pain is poor. A pain score is obtained by measuring from the left-hand end of the line to the mark in millimetres. When scores are obtained at intervals over a period of time a pain profile can be constructed (Fig. 3.3) and this can be used to assess the effects of treatment, or the natural variations in pain throughout each day.

The VAS is easy to use in a clinical setting and it must be completed at the correct times to obtain an accurate record. Difficulties may be encountered in patients who are cognitively impaired by birth, age, or a disease process that affects brain function. In addition, recent work has shown that only a minor-

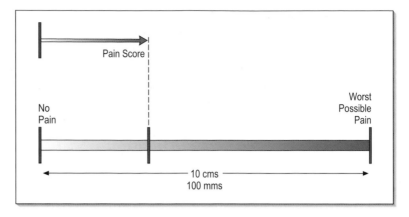

Fig 3.2 The visual analogue scale (VAS) and a recoded pain score.

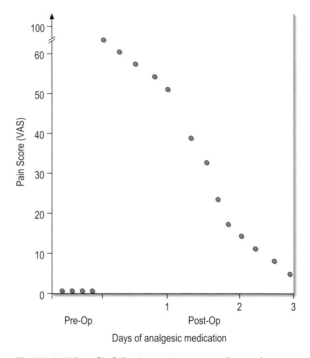

Fig 3.3 A VAS profile following a minor surgical procedure.

ity of patients using the scale at home do so at the times speci-fied by a clinician. The scale has the virtue of transcending the boundaries of language – something that is not always true with verbal scales. In addition, to address this issue the British Pain Society has produced simple pain scales in multiple lan-guages (see their website www.BritishPainSociety.org).

Combined numerical and word-based scales

In its simplest form a verbal scale provides a series of graded descriptions of pain severity, each of which may be given a number. At times the scales are used with an associated numerical scale that implies that changes in levels of pain occur with mathematical precision. This gives a false sense of accuracy, and it is better to rely upon the description of pain severity and the position that it occupies relative to other descriptive terms in a hierarchy of terms. For example, a simple form of the scale would be 'no pain', 'mild pain', 'moderate pain' and 'severe pain'. These terms are unlikely to cause confusion amongst patients, but interpretation can be open to question because the significance of the terms may vary from one person to another. What is important, however, is the patient's own perception of what they feel. The clinician becomes concerned only if there is a gross discrepancy between the observation of the patient's behaviour and the rating made. This may be due to the patient misunderstanding how to use the scale. Such a discrepancy may be an indication of what the sufferer wishes the doctor to conclude about his or her condition; this is important and should not be disregarded. Patients who rate their pain as very severe, when this seems incongruous with the behaviour, may be indicating distress.

In the case of young children, whose ability to describe pain is less well developed, the use of a series of facial expressions is recommended. The Faces Rating Scale is shown in Figure 3.4 – the child is told that face No.1 on the left means that the

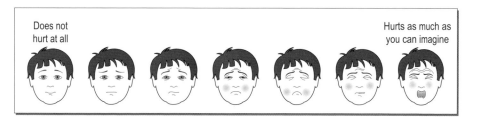

Does not hurt at all   Hurts as much as you can imagine

The use of neutral no pain face and the lack of tears on the worst pain possible face avoid the possibility of confusing pain severity with happiness/sadness.

Faces pain scales have been developed using cartoon faces. These are popular with children and parents but have been shown to be less accurate.

The nurse must explain to the child that the first face represents no hurt at all and that the last face represents as much as they can possibly imagine.

Fig 3.4 Adapted from Glasper E, Richardson J 2005 A textbook of children's and young people's nursing. Elsevier Churchill Livingstone.

condition does not hurt at all, and face No.5 means that it hurts a lot, and the child is asked to choose a face that matches his or her pain.

Pain assessment in neonates is very difficult; several observer-rated behavioural scores are available and these may include facial expression, movement and heart rate. Similar scales have been devised for people with significant cognitive impairment, for example elderly patients with organic brain diseases.

The McGill Pain Questionnaire

Pain experience has dimensions other than severity and in 1975 the McGill Pain Questionnaire (MPQ) was devised based upon three dimensions of pain: the sensory, the affective/motivational, and the cognitive/evaluative. The sensory dimension of pain is concerned with discrimination amongst its sensory qualities, the motivational/affective dimension is concerned with the emotional impact of pain, and the cognitive/evaluative dimension relates past experience to present circumstances.

The full questionnaire proved too long for use in most clinical situations and in 1987 a shorter form was produced (SF-MPQ). The McGill group also developed the 'Present Pain Index' or PPI, a five-part word scale in which the words describing the severity of pain are rated 1–5. The SF-MPQ, with words from the affective and sensory categories of the standard form, together with the PPI and a VAS form a complete test battery. An adapted version of the SF-MPQ is shown in Figure 3.5. Its robustness has been shown by its sensitivity to the assessment of various treatments for pain including analgesics, epidural analgesic blocks and the use of transcutaneous electrical nerve stimulation (TENS). The three scores derived from it are the sum of intensity rank values of words selected from the affective and sensory scales, and the measurements of pain severity by the PPI and the VAS.

Difficulties may arise in the use of the MPQ amongst less well-educated patients who normally do not use the words contained in the scales and, therefore, may have problems in making an appropriate choice to express their own experiences. Alternatively their first language may not be English.

To overcome linguistic problems, the VAS may be used in conjunction with line diagrams of the body that allow the patient to shade areas affected by pain in a manner that indicates both its location and type (pain drawings, see Fig. 3.6). As an alternative, the Faces Rating Scale may be used. The

SHORT-FORM McGILL PAIN QUESTIONNAIRE

PLEASE SELECT FROM THE LIST BELOW WORDS THAT YOU WOULD USE TO DESCRIBE YOUR PAIN
(tick the appropriate box in each column for each word).

		NONE	MILD	MODERATE	SEVERE
Sensory					
Throbbing	1	☐	☐	☐	☐
Shooting	2	☐	☐	☐	☐
Stabbing	3	☐	☐	☐	☐
Sharp	4	☐	☐	☐	☐
Cramping	5	☐	☐	☐	☐
Gnawing	6	☐	☐	☐	☐
Hot-burning	7	☐	☐	☐	☐
Aching	8	☐	☐	☐	☐
Heavy	9	☐	☐	☐	☐
Tender	10	☐	☐	☐	☐
Splitting	11	☐	☐	☐	☐
Affective					
Tiring/exhausting	12	☐	☐	☐	☐
Sickening	13	☐	☐	☐	☐
Fearful	14	☐	☐	☐	☐
Punishing/cruel	15	☐	☐	☐	☐

MARK A CROSS ON THE LINE BELOW TO INDICATE THE INTENSITY OF YOUR PAIN

(a) RIGHT NOW:

No Pain |————————————————————| Worst Possible pain

(b) AT ITS WORST IN THE LAST MONTH

No Pain |————————————————————| Worst Possible pain

(c) AT ITS BEST IN THE LAST MONTH

No Pain |————————————————————| Worst Possible pain

PRESENT PAIN INDEX (PPI)

WHICH OF THE FOLLOWING WORDS EXPLAINS YOUR PRESENT PAIN (tick one only)
Score

0	No Pain	☐
1	Mild Pain	☐
2	Discomforting	☐
3	Distressing	☐
4	Horrible	☐
5	Excruciating	☐

Fig 3.5 Short-form McGill Pain Questionnaire. Adapted with permission from Melzack R 1987 The Short-form McGill Questionnaire. Pain 30:191–197.

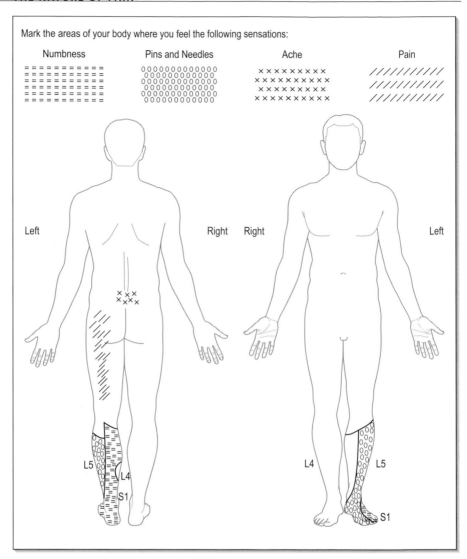

Fig 3.6 A body outline for recording pain qualities. Pain qualities associated with a prolapsed intervertebral disc and nerve root compression at L5–S1. Adapted with permission from Main C & Spanswick CC 2000, Pain management: an interdisciplinary approach. Churchill Livingstone, 2000 p. 133, Fig. 7A1.

development of computer-generated, interactive animations in which the subject relates his or her pain to levels of pressure, heat, and piercing with a needle, using an animated VAS, is a recent and more sophisticated means of assessing pain. The results obtained with this method have been found to correlate with values obtained in the SF-MPQ.

Neuropathic pain scales

Some pain is generated from within the nervous system itself. Such neuropathic pain may be due to peripheral nerve damage (e.g. after trauma) or central nervous system problems (e.g. after stroke). Specific scales have been devised to try to distinguish between nociceptive pain transmitted by the normal pain pathways and neuropathic pain. Such a distinction may help to guide clinical practice and treatment.

Pain drawings

The pain drawing is a form of communication between the patient and the clinician, and it is a practical aid to the location and nature of pain. It may be added to the assessment battery including also results of the VAS, PPI and the SF-MPQ. The diagrams in Figure 3.6 show body outlines on which patients are asked to indicate the site of their pain. Symbols for pains with different qualities increase the information provided. The site and description of pain may be classical for a given pathological condition, for example after a lumbar disc prolapse causing sciatica and sensory changes in the leg. Patterns of pains that do not fit recognized clinical descriptions are useful because they alert the doctor to the possibility that psychological rather than physical factors are the main cause for the pain complaints. In other words, the description given may represent a failure to cope with pain. However, it must be recognized that all pain does not present in a classical dermatomal distribution, for example the pain of complex regional pain syndrome, and that this alone should not lead to the conclusion that there is no physical cause for the pain.

Pain diary

Often patients are asked to keep a diary of daily activities, pain using the PPI and/or VAS, and treatments (Fig. 3.7). This permits monitoring of pain on a daily basis even when patients are at home and away from the observation of the medical team. A diary is often used to establish a baseline of activity, pain and medication prior to the design and implementation of a pain management programme for chronic pain.

Assessment of behaviours

Human behaviour is, by and large, habitual not random. It is actively directed by thoughts and emotions and is subject to modification as a result of intrinsic changes in those functions, and as the result of the effects of the environment upon them. Behaviour associated with illness differs from that of the same

PAIN DIARY

Please describe the type of activity, mood and medication for each hour of a typical day. Use the 0–10 scale for pain and indicate how the pain affects your activity and feelings. Record medication as name and number of tablets.

Time	Pain	Activity	Mood	Medication
6.00am	3	In bed	Slightly low	–
7.00am	8	Up for breakfast	Slightly low	2 tablets Co-proxamol
8.00am	5	Reading	Slightly low	–
9.00am	7	Walking	Anxious	–

Fig 3.7 A pain diary. Recordings made throughout one day by a patient with chronic low back pain.

individual when in a healthy state. For example, acute pain results in grimacing, vocalization, rubbing and perhaps limping, depending upon the nature and site of the pain. Different and more varied patterns are observed in chronic pain states. The illness behaviour is determined by the actual debilitating effects of disease or injury, and a patient's belief in what seems to be its cause and their attitude to it. Behaviour is influenced by the social expectations; for example, it is accepted that illness usually requires a period of rest and time away from school or work and it is expected that sufferers will make every effort to seek treatment to get well again. In addition, once well, they should return to their usual domestic and social activities. These are the sanctions granted by society to its members, and its expectations of them when they become ill. Observation of those who are ill or injured and in pain is an aspect of the clinical investigation of pain (see Ch. 18) because the clinician seeks to determine whether or not the behaviour exhibited is in keeping with what would be expected normally and to determine whether it is exaggerated, or altered in some way, unconsciously or not. Direct observations of the behaviour of patients, therefore, are one form of assessment.

A further aspect of the clinical examination of behaviour involves deciding whether or not it is in keeping with the results of examinations in the consulting room when observed in a different environment (e.g. at home or in the wider community). Do patients, for example, unnecessarily use a walking stick, crutches, wheelchair, or other aids, do they spend more time resting than is necessary, and is their consumption of medication including 'over the counter preparations' in keeping with a clinically judged need?

Finally, the clinician might wish to obtain a record of the patient's daily activities by means of a diary of activities such as walking time and distances, time spent in and out of bed, and social and physical activities undertaken at set times of the day (see Fig. 3.7). Confirmation of this record by a close friend or relative is advised.

Sex, gender and pain

Many laboratory experiments on pain thresholds suggested that women have lower pain thresholds than men for induced pain with modalities such as heat, cold, pressure and electric shock. However, these studies are poor surrogates for pain in a real life setting. There is little evidence that males and females differ significantly in sensitivity to clinical pain. There is no good evidence that there is a gender difference in self-reported pain intensity or unpleasantness. If there is a gender difference then it is probably most important in the later stages of pain processing. Women with pain are more likely than men to continue to experience pain-related mood changes. It is likely that men and women experience different emotional responses to pain and express them differently over time. Several chronic pain problems have a specific sex distribution, and many of these pain syndromes are commoner in women (e.g. headache, migraine, fibromyalgia and back pain). There are also important sex differences in the pharmacokinetics and pharmacodynamics of various analgesic drugs and their side effects (e.g. women experience more nausea than men with opioid analgesics). There is some evidence that women are at greater risk of underprescribing of analgesics.

Race, ethnicity and pain

The clinical pain experience varies across racial and ethnic groups. There is little difference in the sensory discriminative aspect of pain processing; the greatest differences are seen in the emotional measures (e.g. depression and fear). These differences may be based on differences between ethnic groups in the meaning of pain and its likely intrusion into occupational and social roles. There are racial differences in styles of coping with pain and the incidence of negative emotions associated with pain. Although it is vital not to allow racial stereotypes to bias treatment decisions, it is important that ethnic and cultural factors are taken into account when planning pain management. Strategies to address affect and behaviour may be particularly important in some groups; these may have to be tailored to the ethnicity and cultural background of the patient and carers.

Pain in neonates and children

Young children's pain was often neglected in the past, and they were often given inadequate analgesia. It was believed that neonates and young children did not experience pain and stress in the same way as adults owing to their immature nervous system; this is not the case. Measurable responses to painful stimuli that can be reduced by analgesia have been observed in all ages including the neonate. Sensory processing in early life is substantially different from that of the adult. However, there is evidence that, as with adults, there is sensitization of the nervous system after prolonged painful stimuli in children. C-fibre function matures later in children than in adults, and so in early life, central wind-up is more dependent on A-fibre activity. Children have different receptor populations to adults, and this may affect pain mechanisms and the efficacy of some therapies. Untreated pain and injury during development may have long-term effects. Infants who experience pain in early life show altered behavioural responses to pain as they mature. Therefore, pain in children needs careful and specialized assessment using validated tools. Optimal analgesia is important on both humanitarian grounds and to help to prevent the development of problems in later life.

Pain in the elderly

Pain is common in old age, but it is not a normal consequence of ageing; pathology is always involved. There are many morphological and neurochemical changes in the elderly brain that could affect pain perception. Electrophysiological studies show slower central processing of incoming noxious stimuli and reduced cortical activation with increasing age. However, there may also be a parallel decline in function of endogenous pain inhibitory systems. The functional significance of these changes remains to be seen. There is no evidence that ageing per se changes pain intensity or immediate unpleasantness of pain. Older people do report less emotional distress and illness and pain. This can lead to miscommunication between the patient and medical team, such that underlying pathology may be masked by behavioural disturbances. There is no evidence that age alone leads to a difference in a person's ability to cope. Older people have the capacity for both active and passive styles of coping, but with age the trend is towards passive, introspective and mature styles. Elderly patients are more likely to ascribe pain to ageing than to give pain excess attention. However, pain is a significant predictor of poor self-rating of health status in the elderly population, and the latter is a predictor of mortality. Careful assessment and the use of modified assessment tools are vital in the evaluation of elderly patients with pain. Therapies aimed at improving function and that emphasize rehabilitation are important.

Self-assessment questions

3.1 In which of the following situations does the Severe Pain Threshold rise?

a. Acute anxiety
b. Depressive states
c. With relaxation
d. Following treatment with analgesic drugs
e. In those injured in battle

3.2 When assessing the pain experience of a patient living at home with chronic low back pain who wishes to enter a pain rehabilitation programme, which measure(s) of pain severity and behaviour would you use?

Basic mechanisms of pain

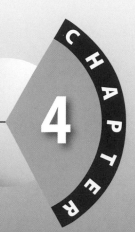

CHAPTER 4

Chapter objectives

After studying this chapter you should be able to:

1 Understand the basic anatomy, physiology and neuropharmacology of normal pain processing.

2 Understand the differences between acute, chronic, nociceptive, and neuropathic pain. Appreciate the differences in pain processing in chronic pain conditions.

3 Understand that pain has psychosocial as well as physical dimensions.

4 Understand that the placebo effect is physiologically and psychologically based.

5 Understand that multimodal therapy is more effective because it targets different aspects of pain processing.

Anatomy, physiology and neuropharmacology of pain

Pain that is perceived after noxious stimuli leads to a series of events in the peripheral nerves, spinal cord and brain (Fig. 4.1).

- Activation of peripheral receptors and primary afferent nociceptive neurons leads to flow of ions through channels in nerve membranes that propagate action potentials. Modification of, and changes in the distribution of, ion channels can occur after peripheral nerve damage; this leads to excitability of these nociceptive neurons.

- Transmission of signals from the periphery occurs, via the dorsal horn of the spinal cord, to the areas of the central nervous system concerned with pain processing.

- Connections are then made to the higher brain centres that are concerned with the perception, affective response and evaluation of pain.

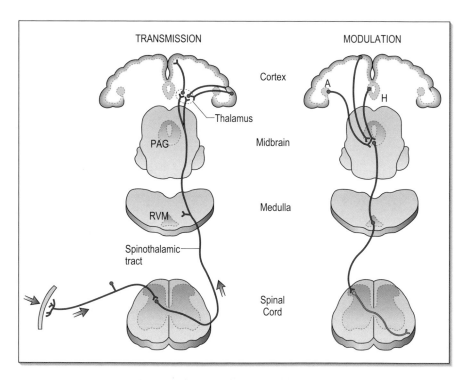

Fig 4.1 Pathways in the spinal and brain cord for pain transmission and modulation. Note that the origin of pain–modulatory pathways includes the cerebral cortex, hypothalamus (H), amygdala (A), periaqeductal grey (PAG), and rostroventral medulla (RVM). From Price DD, Psychological mechanisms of pain & analgesia, Progress in pain research and management, Vol 15. IASP Press 1999, p. 138 Fig. 1.

- The nociceptive pathways are modulated in the spinal cord and brain by a process known as 'gating'; this may act at several levels to inhibit pain transmission.
- The final stage in nociception is pain perception.

Peripheral nociception

Primary afferent nociceptors are classified according to their conduction velocity and size. There are two types of primary afferent nerve fibres involved in somatic nociception:

- Myelinated, thermal and mechanothermal Aδ fibres (conduction velocity 5–30 m/s and diameter 1–5 μm), which cause fast, sharp pain
- Non-myelinated, polymodal heat, chemical and mechanical C fibres (conduction velocity < 3 m/s and diameter < 1.5 μm), which cause slow, burning pain (80% of primary afferent nociceptors).

Peripheral receptors are free nerve endings that are grouped into high threshold mechanoreceptors and polymodal nociceptors. In response to any painful stimulus there is an initial sharp, localized and brief pain called first pain; the receptors responsible for this pain are the high threshold mechanoreceptor (Aδ) fibres. These are distributed over the body surface, muscle and joints. The first pain is followed by second pain, dull, poorly localized and aching pain that lasts beyond the termination of the painful stimulus. The receptors responsible for this pain are polymodal nociceptors (C fibres) and are distributed in most parts of the body including the viscera.

It may be more useful to classify these pathways according to their neurochemical characteristics and spinal connections. Tissue damage releases inflammatory mediators that sensitize nociceptive terminals producing hyperalgesia (increased sensitivity to painful stimuli) and allodynia (pain sensation after non-painful stimuli). Hyperalgesia may occur to pinprick or temperature within the area of nerve injury (primary – from C fibres) or spread more widely (secondary – from dorsal horn or brain). Allodynia may be dynamic, static, punctuate, chemical and temperature provoked or induced by skin stretching. Nociceptors are stimulated by a variety of endogenous agents (e.g. 5-hydroxytryptamine (5-HT), bradykinin, histamine, prostaglandins, substance P). These fibres transmit information to the central nervous system. The cell bodies of the peripheral nerves are in the dorsal root ganglion of the spinal cord, and that of the trigeminal nerve is in the trigeminal ganglion.

Visceral nociception

Chronic visceral pain presents a clinical challenge. The physiology of visceral pain generation and transmission is less well understood than that of somatic pain. The visceral system warns us of internal rather than external damage, so has evolved differently. Visceral pain occurs with distension and ischaemia rather than direct thermal or mechanical trauma. It is often less well localized and referred to the area of organ development; for example testicular pain is referred to the abdomen, and splenic pain is referred to the shoulder.

The viscera are innervated by two sets of primary afferent fibres. These have high threshold receptors that respond to mechanical stimuli and low threshold receptors that encode the magnitude of the stimulus. There are also silent nociceptors that can be sensitized if inflammation occurs. Visceral afferents may become sensitized and respond to stimuli that were previously innocuous. Vagal afferents project to the nucleus of the tractus solitarius from the oesophagus to the transverse colon. The rest of the large bowel is innervated via afferents from the sacral dorsal root ganglia that project centrally via the sacral spinal cord. The gut also has innervation from the splanchnic nerves that project to T5–L2 of the spinal cord. These systems form a major synapse at the coeliac plexus. Visceral afferents form about 10% of the afferent input to the dorsal horn where they pass to laminae I, II, V and X (see below). Therefore, visceral pain is often poorly localized because of the low receptor density. The visceral afferents project to many different central sites (e.g. the spinothalamic, spinohypothalamic, spinosolitary and spinoreticular tracts and dorsal columns). Innocuous gut stimulation can sometimes cause neurotransmitter release and lead to central sensitization and chronic pain.

The pelvic viscera respond to distension or traction with pain signals. There are almost no Aδ fibres in the pelvic viscera. The inferior hypogastric plexus is the main autonomic pelvic relay. The complexity of the nerve supply to pelvic organs makes the diagnosis of pelvic pains difficult.

Hypersensitivity commonly occurs in somatic areas from referred visceral pain; for example abdominal muscle tender points are common in patients with pelvic visceral pain. Viscero-somatic convergence causes these phenomena via changes in neurotransmitters. There is also viscero-visceral hyperalgesia, whereby problems in one organ can generate pain in another viscus.

Spinal processing of pain

Most primary afferent nociceptors enter the spinal cord via the ventrolateral part of the dorsal root; some then travel rostrally or caudally. They synapse with second order neurons in the dorsal horn. The grey matter of the spinal cord is divided into 10 layers (Rexed's laminae); the dorsal horn comprises laminae I–VI. Primary afferent nociceptive fibres terminate in laminae I and II (the substantia gelatinosa). Some Aδ-fibres pass as deep as lamina V. The fibres in the dorsal horn act to regulate the transmission of stimuli to the brain. There are fewer visceral afferent nociceptors, but they are more widely distributed. They do not have the same precision of somatotrophic representation; this explains in part the poor localization of visceral pain. They mainly terminate in laminae I and V; referral of visceral pain to somatic structures may be modulated here.

There are many different neurotransmitters in the dorsal horn, e.g. noradrenaline (norepinephrine), 5–HT, gamma amino butyric acid (GABA), glycine, glutamate, opioids, other peptides, adenosine, capsaicin and cannabinoids. Tissue damage alters the concentration and distribution of the various neurotransmitters in the spinal cord in a way that often outlasts the initiating stimulus (Fig. 4.2). The main excitatory transmitters are glutamate and aspartate and the main inhibitory transmitters are glycine and GABA.

Several ascending pathways transmit nociceptive information to the brain. Although the spinothalamic tract was always considered the most important pathway, this may not be the case in some chronic pain conditions. The spinothalamic tract lies anterolaterally in the spinal cord white matter. It projects to the thalamus, periaqueductal grey matter, reticular formation and hypothalamus. The spinoreticular pathway transmits pain signals; it originates in deeper spinal cord laminae and terminates in the reticular formation of the brainstem. It then projects to the thalamus and other central sites. Other pathways subserving visceral pain transmission may be involved in modulation of afferent pain signals and activating descending inhibitory pathways.

Sympathetic nervous system and pain

The sympathetic nervous system may play an important role in pain processing and the generation of persistent pain after trauma; for example after a peripheral nerve injury, neuromas may form that involve sympathetic fibres. Peripheral sympathetic fibres may also sprout and migrate into areas that are

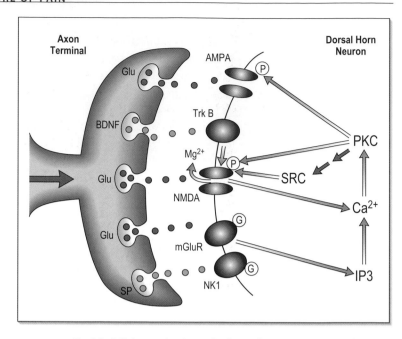

Fig 4.2 Cellular mechanisms of enhanced synaptic activity in the spinal dorsal horn after injury. BDNF = brain-derived neurotrophic factor; G = G-protein; Glu = glutamate; IP3 = inosital triphosphate; mGluR = metabotropic glutamate receptor; NK1 = neurokinin-1 receptor; P = phosphorylation; PKC = protein kinase C; SP = substance P; trk = tyrosine kinase B receptor. From Dubner R & Ren K, Brainstem modulation of pain after inflammation. In: Villaneuva L, Dickenson AH & Ollat H The pain system in normal and pathological states: a primer for clinicians, Progress in pain research and management, Vol 31. IASP Press 2004 as for Fig 4.1.

not normally supplied by these autonomic fibres. These ectopic fibres form links with regenerating sensory nerves and cause pain; various neurotransmitters are involved (e.g. substance P). There may also be coupling of sympathetic and afferent nociceptive fibres in the dorsal root ganglion after trauma, with increased release of noradrenaline (norepinephrine) and upregulation of adrenoceptors leading to pain. This means that the receptor population changes and its sensitivity to agonists increases (Fig. 4.3). The involvement of the sympathetic nervous system in clinical pain conditions is supported by the fact that sympathectomy may be a useful therapy in some cases.

Pain processing in the brain

The dorsal horn of the spinal cord sends projections to various brain areas, e.g. lateral thalamus, medial thalamus; these then

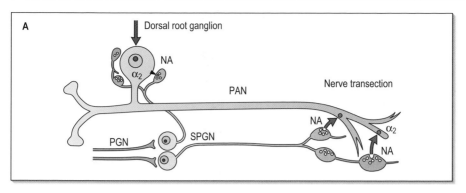

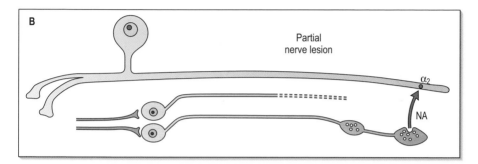

Fig 4.3 The influence of sympathetic activity and catecholamines on primary afferent neurons (PAN). (A) Nerve transection. The sympathetic-afferent interaction is located in the neuroma and in the dorsal root ganglion. It is mediated by noradrenaline (norepinephrine) (NA) released from sympathetic postganglionic neurons (SPGN) and by α2-adrenoceptors expressed at the plasma membrane of afferent neurons. PGN, preganglionic neuron. (B) Partial nerve lesion. Partial nerve injury is followed by a decrease of the sympathetic innervation density (stippled sympathetic postganglionic neuron), which induces an upregulation of functional α2-adrenoceptors at the membrane of intact afferent fibres. From Baron R & Jänig W, The role of the sympathetic nervous system. In: Villaneuva L, Dickenson AH & Ollat H The pain system in normal and pathological states: a primer for clinicians, Progress in pain research and management, Vol 31. IASP Press 2004 as for Fig 4.1.

relay to multiple areas in the somatosensory cortex (Fig. 4.4). However, it has now been shown that the thalamus is not the only important area for pain processing. Areas of the brain that may be important in pain processing are the periaqueductal grey matter, insula and the cingulate cortex. A variety of lesions within the brain can cause pain; the thalamus is particularly important, especially its reticulothalamic projections. Recent advances in functional brain imaging have allowed better

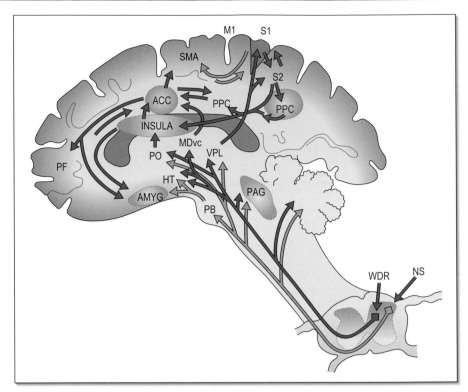

Fig 4.4 A diagram of ascending pathways, subcortical studies and cerebral cortical structures involved in processing pain. ACC = anterior cingulate cortex; PO = posterior nuclear complex; AMYG = amygdala; HT = hypothalamus; M1 = primary motor area; MDvc = ventrocaudal part of medial dorsal nucleus; NS = nociceptive specific; PAG = periaqueductal grey; PB = parabrachial nucleus of the dorsolateral pons; PCC = posterior cingulate cortex; PF = prefrontal cortex; PPC = posterior parietal complex; S1, S2 = first and second somatosensory cortical areas; SMA = supplementary motor area; VPL = ventroposterior lateral nucleus; WDR = wide dynamic range. From Price DD & Bushnell MC. Pain dimensions in psychological methods of pain control: basic science and clinical perspectives, Progress in pain research and management, Vol 29. IASP 2004 as for Fig 4.1.

understanding of the role of higher centres in nociception. Some of the psychological aspects of pain appreciation and behaviour have now been elucidated using imaging such as positron emission tomography (PET) and functional magnetic resonance imaging (fMRI). Different levels in the central nervous system modulate the pain experience; they also play a role in phenomena such as the placebo response, hypnosis and distraction. Functional brain imaging has enhanced the understanding of the essential role of higher centres in pain perception.

Modulation of pain processing by 'gating'

Tissue injury does not always lead to perception of pain, e.g. soldiers injured in battle do not always report pain from their wounds. Therefore, the nervous system has 'gating' mechanisms that can modify the passage of pain signals and the perception of pain (see Fig. 1.3). This 'gating' of pain signals can occur at many levels including the dorsal horn of the spinal cord and the brain. The output from the dorsal horn of the spinal cord depends on the input from the periphery, regulatory neurons in the spinal cord and descending projections from the brain (gating). The nociceptive neurons in the spinal cord are modulated by input from non-nociceptive, myelinated Aβ afferents. Opening or closing of the 'gate' is dependent on the relative activity in the large diameter (Aβ) and small diameter fibres (Aδ and C), with activity in the large diameter fibres tending to close the 'gate' and activity in the small diameter fibres tending to open it. Pain impulses can pass through only when the gate is open, and not when it is closed. Therefore, if nociceptive input exceeds Aβ-fibre input, then the gate is open and the pain impulse ascends the spinal cord to the brain. If Aβ-fibre input exceeds nociceptive input then the gate is closed and the pain impulse is stopped or diminished owing to the action of the inhibitory neurotransmitters and, therefore, does not pass up the spinal cord. Hence rubbing the skin activates Aβ afferent, myelinated, fast-conducting fibres, and can switch off pain transmission. An essential part of the theory is that the brain's descending inhibitory system influences the position of the 'gate'. There are neurochemical mechanisms in the spinal cord that act as a 'filter' for pain signalling to the brain; for example opioids may be involved in spinal pain modulation (Fig. 4.5). Persistent pain can be self-generating. Prolonged C-fibre activation alters the pattern of gene transcription in the dorsal root ganglion and dorsal horn cells. This causes increased expression of pain-related neurotransmitters (e.g. capsaicin). The dorsal horn neurons are modulated by projections from the brain that arise in the pons and medulla that are probably mediated via noradrenaline (norepinephrine) and 5-HT.

Acute, chronic, nociceptive and neuropathic pain

The description of the physiology of pain given above is an oversimplification of what is a very complex process. The nervous system is plastic and it changes in response to stimuli.

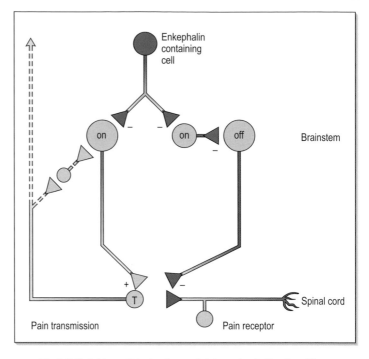

Fig 4.5 Opioid-mediated pain-modulatory circuit. Reprinted by permission of the publisher from 'Gedanken Experiment' by Howard L Fields and Donald D Price in the *Placebo Effect*: an Interdisciplinary Exploration, edited by Anne Harrington, p 99, Cambridge, Mass: Harvard University Press, Copyright © 1997 by the President and Fellows of Harvard College 1997.

Repeated nociceptive barrages may result in the nervous system becoming sensitized – this is sometimes termed 'wind-up'. In this situation, normally non-noxious stimuli may become painful and pain signals may be generated without any noxious input. Therefore, in chronic pain there is aberrant peripheral pain processing, as well as abnormal pain pathways in the spinal cord and brain, and psychological maladaptations and behaviours in response to unremitting pain.

The pain that most of us experience in everyday life is nociceptive owing to stimulation of normal Aδ and C-fibre polymodal nociceptors. This acute pain acts as a useful warning (e.g. pain after brief trauma, inflammation or surgery). Its duration is usually relatively brief, and it resolves with tissue healing and time. Chronic pain is different because it outlasts the original stimulus. Sometimes the inciting event that triggers chronic pain is difficult to identify. This type of pain does not warn of tissue damage and it serves no useful purpose. It is often accompanied by behavioural and mood changes because it is prolonged and usually outside the person's normal pain experience. There are several psychological risk factors for the development of chronic pain. Cognitive variables such as fear-avoidance beliefs are often important.

Neuropathic pain is different to nociceptive pain. It is initiated, or caused, by a primary lesion or dysfunction in the nervous system. It is commoner in older people. The population prevalence is about 1%, and neuropathic pain comprises about 25% of all referrals to chronic pain clinics in the UK. It has different qualities and tends to persist. The diagnosis of neuropathic pain is made by careful clinical history and examination including somatosensory function. There are validated scales to assess neuropathic pain. Treatments should be mechanism and not syndrome based.

Peripheral nerve damage leads to long-term changes in the central nervous system that can lead to persistent pain (e.g. phantom limb pain or peripheral neuropathy). Some pain conditions can arise from damage within the spinal cord (e.g. pain from multiple sclerosis or transverse myelitis) or within the brain (e.g. pain after stroke). A cascade of neurochemical changes follow damage to the nervous system that results in a sensitization of neural elements involved in the processing of noxious information. The nervous system is plastic; new circuits are constantly being formed and broken at all levels of the neural pathway. Peripheral nerve damage may result in areas of demyelination that alter nerve transmission and lead to aberrant conduction and hyperexcitability. Hyperalgesia and allodynia are typically present in neuropathic pain. A fibres are often selectively lost distal to the damaged nerve and neuronal death occurs in the dorsal root ganglia; this all leads to pain. Reinnervation is stimulated, but C fibres may join to low threshold cutaneous sensory fibres and cause persistent pain. Small fibre afferents may expand over large areas, causing hyperalgesia and neuropathic pain. Activity occurs in axonal sprouts, demyelinated nerves and dorsal ganglia without stimulation, so patients complain of spontaneous shooting and burning pain. This is sometimes coupled with a local inflammatory reaction to nerve damage. The autonomic nervous system may become involved if sympathic fibres form links with damaged dorsal root ganglia; thus, some neuropathic pain has a sympathetic component. Although there are many different mechanisms that can lead to neuropathic pain, its clinical presentation can be variable; this leads to difficulties in assessing and managing neuropathic pain.

Psychological aspects of pain

Pain of any kind is associated with sensory and emotional components and the desire to end the experience or escape. The initial phase in the pain experience is sensory-discriminative input from nociceptors; this stage involves limited cognitive processing. When pain persists, there is an affective response to its long-term implications; this can be thought of in a wider context as suffering. This extended pain affect is based on complex cognitive processes; these may include reflection on the meaning of pain and its interference with normal daily life (see Ch. 5). The final phase in pain modulation is the behavioural response to pain with activity modification. This behaviour aspect of chronic pain is an important target for management strategies. It is possible to address the way that people deal with pain, their cognitive processing and their attributions about what pain means (see Ch. 18).

The placebo response

Investigation of the placebo response has given insights into the biological mechanisms that modulate nociception. The placebo response is the effect that follows the administration of an inert medical treatment. A reduction in symptoms results from factors related to the subject's perception of the therapeutic intervention. The therapeutic context is a critical factor in this response. The placebo response occurs because the global experience of pain may be increased or decreased by complex modulation at supraspinal levels. Many factors influence this higher processing, for example emotion, attention, stress, fear, anticipation, distraction and mood. When a patient is experiencing pain, then the perception that an effective treatment has been given may be sufficient to produce significant analgesia. Conditioning and suggestion also influence pain by inducing expectations. The memory of past pain experiences also influences the placebo response. There is no single mechanism for the placebo; it occurs via different pathways. Placebo analgesia has been shown by functional brain imaging to result in decreased neural activity in the pain-processing areas of the brain, for example the thalamus, and anterior insular and cingulate cortex. The response is partly mediated by endogenous neurotransmitters, for example non-opioid mediators, opioids, β-adrenergic systems and 5-HT.

Multimodal therapies

Pain processing is therefore complex, and this has important implications for pain management. Many different physical and psychological strategies can be used alone or in parallel with other therapies for dealing with acute and chronic pain. In complex pain problems, it is unlikely that a simple, single strategy will be very effective. It is important to adopt a multiprofessional approach to assessment, investigation and management of complex pain problems. Multimodal treatment that targets different parts of the pain pathways is the logical way to manage all pain.

Self-assessment questions

Answer 'True' or 'False' to the following statements:

4.1 Peripheral nociceptors:

   a. Are myelinated fibres that conduct at less than 3 m/s

   b. Are unmyelinated fibres with a diameter of less than 1.5 μm

   c. Are nerve endings that are high threshold mechanoreceptors and polymodal nociceptors

   d. Enter the spinal cord via the ventrolateral part of the dorsal root

   e. Synapse in layer VI of the dorsal horn

4.2 Visceral structures:

   a. Are innervated by two sets of primary afferent fibres

   b. May become sensitized and respond to stimuli that were previously innocuous

   c. Are supplied by vagal afferents that project to the nucleus of the tractus solitarius from the oesophagus to the descending colon

   d. Have innervation from the splanchnic nerves that project to T5–T12 of the spinal cord

   e. Project to many different central sites

4.3 The main excitatory transmitters in the spinal cord are:

   a. Glutamate

   b. Aspartate

   c. Glycine

   d. GABA

   e. Opioids

4.4 The placebo response:

    a.   Is the effect that follows the administration of an active medical treatment

    b.   Is due to factors related to the subject's perception of the therapeutic intervention

    c.   Is affected by emotion

    d.   Results from a single mechanism

    e.   Has no physiological basis

The biopsychosocial nature of pain

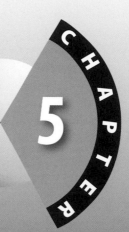

CHAPTER 5

Chapter objectives

After studying this chapter you should be able to:

1 Describe basic concepts of personality, cognition, emotion and pain-related behaviour.

2 Understand the importance of pain, and patients and carers' attitudes towards, and beliefs about, the causes of pain. Understand the role that their beliefs about their ability to cope with and control pain have on the outcome. Appreciate the important contribution families, carers, healthcare professionals and society make to the development and maintenance of pain.

3 Apply your knowledge to the psychological analysis and understanding of acute and chronic pain conditions.

4 Understand the nature and role of psychological, social and employment issues in the transition from acute to chronic pain.

5 Draw up an outline of the main psychological resources needed as a basis for a pain management programme.

Psychological aspects of pain experience

Consideration of the sensory aspects of pain alone does not encompass the contributions made to the experience by emotions and cognitive processes. Pain arises as the result of parallel and interconnected activities in specific areas of the brain. Sensory inputs act to generate cognitive activity, including memory functions, the emotions, motor responses and complex behaviours patterns. The original Gate Theory concept has been expanded to show how areas of the brain concerned with sensation, cognition and emotion might interact centrally and modulate the flow of neuronal activity in the spinal cord due to noxious stimulation (Fig. 5.1). To understand the complexities involved it is helpful to look at each function in turn.

A burn of the skin of the hand gives rise to noxious stimulation that is recorded centrally in the sensory cortex and a reflex motor response leading to withdrawal of the hand as a result of a spinal reflex. At the same time awareness of the burn evokes memories of past similar events and an associated

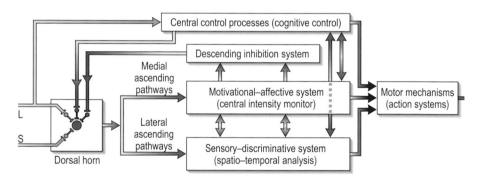

Fig 5.1 The Gate control theory extended. The output of the T cell in the dorsal horn projects to the sensory–discriminative system via the lateral ascending system and to the motivational–affective system via the medial ascending system. A heavy line running from the large fibre system to the central controll processes in the brain represents the central control 'trigger', composed of the dorsal column and the dorsolateral projection systems. These project back to the dorsal horn as well as to the sensory–discriminative and the motivational–affective systems. The brainstem inhibitory control system is activated by impulses in the medial descending system and provides descending control on the dorsal horn. There is interaction between the motivational–affective and the sensory–discriminative systems as indicated by the arrows. The net effect of all these interacting systems is activation of the motor (action) system. Reproduced with permission from Melzack & Casey, The Skin Senses edited by DR Kenshalo 1968. Charles C Thomas Publisher Ltd, Springfield, Illinois, USA.

sense of unpleasantness indicates activation of the emotional cortex. After the initial withdrawal from the hot surface the person usually behaves in a way that minimizes the burning sensation/pain (e.g. by holding the hand under cold water). In other words, in this simple example a judgement based upon knowledge and past experience results in a form of behaviour designed to minimize injury and pain.

In the more complex disorder of acute appendicitis, pain is located in the abdomen. Cognitive processes result in an emotional change, usually anxiety, and a complex set of behaviours aimed at gaining information about the reason for the pain and finding a means of relief. The behaviour pattern exhibited by the subject is the result of cognitive activities and is known as the coping mechanism (the way of dealing with pain). These mechanisms reflect, in part, the individual's cultural, social and family background. In the case of chronic pain problems, for example low back pain, the pain of arthritic diseases or of cancer, there are even greater variations in emotional and behaviour patterns and coping responses. The further we move away from a simple acute pain disorder towards chronic pain states, the more complex the cognitive, emotional, behavioural and social elements become (Box 5.1).

The biopsychosocial model

The definition of pain makes it clear that both biological and psychological factors are part of the experience of pain. The influence of social factors completes the three elements of what is known as the 'biopsychosocial model'. In the analysis of pain problems, especially those that are chronic, all three aspects overlap and must be considered (Fig. 5.2).

Box 5.1

Acute and chronic pain: associated emotion and behaviour

- Acute and chronic pain give rise to different physical and emotional behavioural responses.

- Acute pain generates anxiety, an associated pattern of autonomic arousal and rapid relief-directed behaviour.

- Chronic pain generates complex and varying patterns of emotion, often with negative emotions that may be associated with maladaptive behaviours and depression.

Fig 5.2 A diagrammatic representation of the biological, psychological and social factors which combine in the biopsychological model of illness. The extent to which the three factors interact will vary within and between individuals.

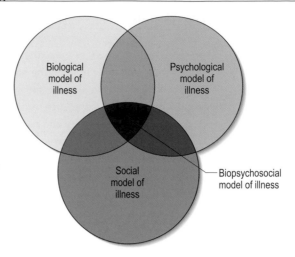

Basic psychological concepts

Personality

Personality can be regarded as each person's emotional and behavioural 'signature' and, although we are unique with respect to our combination of personality traits, there are common elements in the range of characteristics shown by the general population. These were recognized centuries ago; for example Hippocrates linked personality characteristics to aspects of bodily function in terms that are still used sometimes to describe mood; for example choleric – hot tempered, and melancholic – depressed or gloomy, refer to opposite mood states. The words used are based upon the role that was once thought to be played by bile in the functions of the human body and mind. In the 20th century Sheldon proposed that body types are linked to certain personality characteristics. For example, he said that the endomorph has a slim build and a quiet nature, the ectomorph in contrast is rounded and jolly, whereas the mesomorph is muscular and well developed, with a personality placed between that of the ectomorph and the endomorph. Both Hippocrates and Sheldon were using a psychosomatic model. In other words they linked features of body structure to mental function. However, those conceptual systems do not have any practical significance now in the understanding of pain, or the management of pain.

Specific theories of personality

Sigmund Freud developed a theory of personality linked to his psychoanalytic theory that was based on the premise that emotion and behaviour are influenced by the unconscious mind. That, he said, is accessible through the interpretation of dreams and memories of early life experiences using a technique known as free association. Freud proposed three components of personality. The ego is the conscious mind and it is in contact with the everyday world, the id is basic, primitive and childlike and the super ego, which is often equated with conscience, exerts control over the id and balances its activity with that of the ego. These concepts are mentalistic and elegant, but do not have an obvious connection with the physiological function of the brain. Certain therapists, however, find Freud's constructs of mental life useful in their areas of counselling and psychotherapy. Freudian concepts led also to the description by Engel of the 'pain-prone personality', the main characteristics of which were described earlier.

In the early years of the 20th century the concept of psychosomatic disorders developed as an extension of the Freudian system. It was argued that certain emotions, or forms of unconscious emotional conflict, are linked to the development of specific disease states that were therefore termed 'psychosomatic'. For example, until quite recently it was believed that the 'type A personality' typified by the restless, ambitious, outgoing workaholic, was especially prone to myocardial infarction, but this has not proved to be the case. In the 1960s, when the psychosomatic approach to personality was losing ground as an explanatory system for diseases such as asthma, hypertension, migraine, peptic ulcer, ulcerative colitis and myocardial infarction, one theory of personality was published that did have some scientific credence, though relatively little practical application to clinical pain management.

Hans Eysenk, a psychologist, defined three major axes for personality traits that he said had a genetic basis; the two of relevance to pain are introversion–extroversion and neuroticism–stability. Recent studies seem to support such a basis for one of them: neuroticism. In addition, recent work has revealed that genes exist in the amygdala, the area of the brain associated with the generation of emotions including anxiety, that seem to be responsible for the ease with which a person becomes anxious (i.e. has a bias towards neuroticism) or tends to remain calm when under pressure.

Two aspects of Eysenk's personality constructs have a link to complaint behaviour and levels of pain amongst individuals with chronic pain. Extraverts complain of pain, whereas introverts are much less likely to do so. Such behaviour in North European cultures where complaints about pain, especially

Box 5.2

Cognitive and emotional factors important in chronic pain states

- The main cognitive factors determining whether a person develops and recovers from disability in chronic painful conditions are their attitudes towards, and beliefs about, their pain and its cause and their prospects for recovery.

- Positive attitudes and beliefs, a good understanding of the nature of pain and its cause and a set of positive beliefs about being able to cope with pain enable positive adaptation to pain and disability.

- Negative attitudes, poor information or understanding and a low level of self-efficacy increase maladaptive behaviours and disability, produce depression and increase pain.

- The concepts described are the basis for psychological programmes of cognitive/behavioural therapy for chronic pain sufferers.

amongst men, are regarded as a sign of 'weakness' might be seen as a disadvantage for the extravert. Individuals who score highly for neuroticism and become anxious easily tend to show anxiety when in pain and to experience more pain than those who have low scores. If a high level of neuroticism is accompanied by extraversion the result is 'an anxious complainer'.

Pain and cognition

Information reaching us from our environment, whether external or internal, is automatically assessed against our existing beliefs and attitudes about any stimulus, for example pain. Next, thoughts, emotions, and actions (behaviours), are generated together with expectations about the outcome of those actions. The act of assessment or appraisal constitutes what is called a 'cognition' in the language of psychology (Box 5.2). The behaviour that emerges from cognitive appraisal, with its emotional colouring, tends to follow a pattern developed or learned in previous similar situations. A knowledge of a sufferer's attitudes, beliefs and the coping mechanisms that stem from them, is an essential part of the psychological management of pain disorders and deliberate attempts are made in management programmes to change all three to enable positive coping strategies to emerge.

Attitudes, expectancies and beliefs

The cognitive factors active in pain states and the development of disability include:

1 Attitudes and beliefs

2 Expectancies about outcome

3 Beliefs about self-efficacy, i.e. ability to cope with and control pain.

There are differences between different individuals' attitudes to, and beliefs about, pain for any given disorder and in each person they influence the perception of symptoms. Negative attitudes and beliefs lead to non-adaptive coping, greater pain and suffering, and greater disability, whereas positive attitudes evoke the opposite response.

Misinterpretation by a person of the extent to which symptoms can be relieved or controlled, and about the outcome of the injury or illness if seen as poor or hopeless, results in negative beliefs. This is known as cognitive distortion, or cognitive error. In its strongest form it is an exaggerated type of loss of self-efficacy that has been described as 'catastrophizing'. This process is linked with the presence of high pain levels, low tolerance for pain, increased disability and the onset of depression. Negative beliefs about pain and its treatment lead pain sufferers to feel that hurt indicates harm, and that because pain reduces physical functioning they face inevitable physical deterioration in the future. This results in demoralization and debilitation. As a result, sufferers avoid activities that they believe will increase pain, become physically deconditioned, that is disabled, and socially increasingly isolated. Patients who have reached this state pose significant management problems.

The term 'self-efficacy' reflects the extent of people's belief that they will be able to control their pain. A high level of self-efficacy correlates with lower levels of pain, less distress, successful treatment and less disability. In contrast, a reduced or absent sense of self-efficacy and negative thinking is associated with a feeling of inability to control pain and the development of depression of mood. Those with low levels of self-efficacy tend to have low pain tolerance and greater need for medication. Therefore, the extent to which individuals believe, or perceive, that they, and/or others, are able to control their pain is a critical factor in determining whether or not perceptions result in positive or negative adaptation. It is clear that negative beliefs are powerful factors in the generation of poor adjustment to pain and the development of long-term disability.

Coping styles and strategies

Coping is a process in which people employ cognitive and behavioural actions to manage specific external/internal demands that are viewed as taxing or exceeding their resources. Individuals have their own coping styles and strategies for coping with pain.

There are those who confront the problems they face in life and work out positive ways of solving or adapting to them; they are regarded as 'copers'. In contrast, there are those who do not cope well and find ways of avoiding situations that provoke pain; these are 'non-copers'. Those who exhibit active or adaptive strategies may, for example, take exercise, and reduce their rest and their dependency on drugs. They attempt to live as normal a life as possible in the presence of pain.

Maladaptive behaviour occurs when there is increasing limitation of physical activity, and social withdrawal, with the level of disability being out of keeping with the level of any demonstrable underlying physical pathology. Those who adopt a passive or non-adaptive strategy from the beginning tend to rest excessively, rely on medication and place control in the hands of others. They suffer from depression more often, especially when they show high levels of passivity and of pain. The role of the pain clinician is to dismantle poor coping strategies and, if possible, to replace them with adaptive ones.

Emotions

Emotions are transient subjective experiences that include the following elements – physiological responses, facial expressions, and a belief that a particular situation is positive or negative. In general we tend to talk about emotions as changes in mood that vary considerably in degree, for example from anxiousness to panic, from mild anger to hate, and minor feelings of low mood to severe depression. Alterations in mood may fall within what is regarded as the normal range; that is a generally acceptable alteration not regarded as illness, beyond which exist abnormal states that are defined as illness. They cause distress and reduction in, or loss of, personal, family, occupational and social functioning. Each change in mood is accompanied by physical changes, especially in the body's autonomic nervous system. For example, acute anxiety results in palpitations, a dry mouth, stomach churning, sweating and pupillary dilation. Changes associated with chronic pain states tend to be towards feelings of depression, although episodes of anxiety do occur at times.

Theories of emotion   There are several theories of emotion linking the physical state and psychological dimensions. By what means, therefore, do changes in bodily and mental activities occur and in what sequence? An early theory (James–Langer) stated that bodily responses to a stimulus precede the experience of emotion, for example a fast heart rate and a trembling hand result in a perception that leads to the emotion of fear. An alternative view (Cannon–Bard) was that perception of a stimulus that gives rise to anxiety or fear occurs independently of physical reactions. A third alternative (Schacter–Singer), which seems to fit common experience more closely, is that the perception of an external stimulus causes physical and psychological arousal involving cognitive processes, an analysis of the significance of the stimulus to the individual and the generation of emotion. Therefore, the change in mood depends upon the person's appraisal of the stimulus, which calls into play memory of past pain experiences involving cultural and family influences.

We believe that noxious stimulation leads to cognitive appraisal of its cause. The significance to the person leads to the development of the emotional component of pain and a particular pattern of behaviour.

The concept of   In present day society the use of the term 'stress' is extremely
emotional stress   common. At times, it seems to be a modern disease that society has imposed upon itself. In fact, stress is not a new experience for man. It is defined as a process that places greater demands on individuals than they can bear, and as a result their capacity to cope is severely stretched or exceeded. All of us become stressed at times, but resistance to becoming stressed, or the ability to bear pressure, varies greatly between individuals and within the same individuals in differing circumstances.

Stress may be acute or chronic. Signs of acute stress are bio-chemical, physiological, cognitive, emotional and behavioural. The overwhelming feeling of the stressed person is a lack of control over events and a sense of helplessness. Persistent feel-ings of helplessness and hopelessness are highly correlated with the development of depression. However, before that stage is reached the individual may appear to have developed a means of coping with persistent stress. With relentless pres-sure, though (overwork is perhaps the most common form in present day life), the individual's health, both physical and emotional, breaks down. A popular term for this process is 'burn-out'. In medical professionals, burn-out is characterized by the following criteria – emotional exhaustion, a low sense of personal accomplishment (despite increasing hours of work), with the collapse of self-esteem and any desire for success, and failure to cope emotionally. This is associated with a sense of detachment from others, and to the development of a cynical attitude towards them, even if they are patients.

The most satisfactory model for the development of stress is one that is based upon the interaction between individuals and their environment or, alternatively, the development of stress internally as a result of personal expectations, beliefs, attitudes and emotions.

Coping with stress, the subject of many book, newspaper and magazine articles, depends fundamentally on 'mediating factors'. They include having a confidante with whom problems may be discussed freely and non-judgmentally, necessary alterations in beliefs and attitudes, changing perceptions to render stressors less threatening, and developing an altered and positive coping style. This may involve individuals reducing their working hours, taking more exercise, recognizing their limits and limiting their expectations to reasonable levels. Therefore, many stresses may be overcome by positive changes in lifestyle, but others, including the presence of pain and other symptoms due to disease or injury, may not be overcome completely leaving residual stress that has to be managed.

Anxiety   Anxiety is an emotion that is experienced by all at some time as a reaction to the stresses of everyday life. When a person needs to produce the best of their mental or physical capabilities (e.g. in the role of actor, taking part in examinations, or a sporting contest), anxiety levels rise; this is a necessary and normal reaction for a good performance. Too high a level of anxiety, however, is unpleasant and counterproductive. Anxious people show changes in thinking, in their physical state and in their behaviour. Internal appraisal by such individuals of their position, with the thought that something unpleasant could happen, triggers anxiety and a range of bodily changes occur if the level of anxiety is sufficiently high. They include sweating, an increased heart rate, dizziness, nausea, tightening of the throat and perhaps loosening of the bowel. We may be able to control anxiety, indicating that we are able to function normally though anxious, and this represents a positive adaptation. However, the experience may result in avoidance behaviour. This means that an event giving rise to anxiety is avoided (e.g. an interview, or an examination). The use of alcohol or drugs may become a means of combating anxiety. These are maladaptive behaviours and may need to become the subject of psychologically based treatment.

If the circumstances in which pain occurs seem to be a significant threat to the life of the person, or carry the prospect of long-term disability, anxiety will be generated. If physical activity causes an increase in, or recurrence of pain, fear of pain may develop. In chronic pain states the fear of provoking pain is a potent cause of prolonged disability and requires treatment.

Pain often provokes anxiety, especially when the cause is unknown, or when a clear diagnosis is not provided. Anxiety occurs in association with acute pain. It occurs also in chronic pain states, when sudden changes in symptoms are experienced, the significance of which is not understood or are feared, or when treatments lose their effect.

In contrast, pain may arise as a result of increased anxiety or emotional tension in common conditions including migraine, tension headaches and episodes of muscle spasm involving particularly the neck and back. In these circumstances the cause of anxiety requires treatment in its own right to eliminate pain. It should be remembered that a sudden increase of pain in cancer sufferers could be due to anxiety, a change in the physical state of the patient, or both.

Depression   Low mood is a common and usually transient experience. Affected individuals feel tired; they lose interest in activities of daily life, and find difficulty in concentrating on reading or watching television programmes. It may affect their ability to cope with their job. Over short periods of time, for example during grief, or after a failure in life (not passing an examination, or not obtaining a sought-after job), such feelings tend to be short lived and can be expected, normally, to lead to only a brief interruption in daily activity. They are not regarded as illness but understandable reactions to adverse situations, particularly those involving loss. Progressive deepening of the mood, with loss of the normal sleep pattern, feelings of guilt and alterations in the mental state, including thoughts of self-harm, indicate a depressive disorder that requires medical treatment (see Ch. 12).

Depression of mood is a characteristic of chronic rather than acute pain. It may be attributed to persistent pain not responding to different treatments and it reflects the failure of treatment and/or of the individual's ability to cope with symptoms of a chronic or a progressive disease. It is associated especially with feelings of loss of control, helplessness and hopelessness. Treatment involves the use of antidepressant medication or psychological techniques, or both.

Those in pain who are depressed usually attribute their feelings to the fact that they are in pain; in some cases, however, the pain may be a major symptom of a depressive illness.

Fear Fear is a specific form of anxiety in which a mild to overwhelming sense or feeling of danger to the self or others is experienced. It is a well-recognized feature of illness and injury and the use of reassurance to dispel it is an important feature of the work of all clinicians. Painful disorders are potential generators of fears, of which there are several that can be readily identified. They include fear of the disease or injury, of pain and disability, of treatment – especially surgery, of loss of earnings and of changes in relationships. There is often a fear that pain will not be adequately controlled. The presence of such negative thoughts is a source of increased pain, decreased activity, increased disability and depression. Therefore, it is important to identify and dispel patients' fears and, of those, fear of pain coupled with avoidance of activity is particularly important. These are strongly related to disability and loss of working ability.

Anger References to anger in illness in general, and pain states in particular, are not often found in the literature. Anger, fear and sadness occur in chronic pain and these are significant predictors of later depression. Anger is a disturbance of mood ranging from a mild irritation to outright physical aggression focused on one or more aspects of a person's life and usually directed at others. For example, anger may develop because people's well-being and ability to pursue their family, social and working life in the usual way has been significantly impaired. Often people speak of their frustrations, rather than their anger, with a painful condition as though it is not a part of themselves, but something alien. In other words the anger is with the illness or injury or the perceived cause of either. Anger may be directed at those providing care – most commonly doctors who are seen as having the power to heal and to control symptoms, but who are seen as not fulfilling those obligations. Anger leads to difficulties in personal interactions and especially with close relatives. It is expressed as irritability that may lead to arguments and to verbal or even physical abuse. All doctors and other clinicians should be aware of, and be prepared to deal with, anger, frustration and resentment arising from painful disorders or illnesses because, as causes of increased emotional tension, they increase pain and reduce the individual's capacity to cope. Such behaviour may alienate family, friends, and healthcare professionals and thus remove potential sources of support even further.

Pain and behaviour

Behaviour changes when we are ill, and illness behaviour refers to the way we think, feel and act in any illness including those that are painful. Illness results in adaptation of our behaviour to it, for example when we take appropriate rest, seek help, accept treatment or express the expectation that we will recover. Non-adaptive behaviours include resting more than is necessary, withdrawing unnecessarily from household and social activities when we could continue them albeit in a modified way, and perhaps going from doctor to doctor seeking ever more investigation and complex treatments. Such behaviour forms the basis of what is termed 'abnormal illness behaviour'. This becomes significant when there is a discrepancy between objective signs of physical abnormality and the presence of inappropriate forms of behaviour. Changes in thinking and mood associated with altered behaviour are dealt with elsewhere in this chapter.

The observation of maladaptive behaviours in painful illnesses led to the development in the late 1960s and early 1970s of a treatment designed to correct them using the technique known as operant conditioning. Psychologists developed it early in the 20th century and it is based upon evidence that all behaviour is influenced by its consequences, which may be either positive or negative, and by the context in which it occurs.

The fundamental element in the operant-conditioning model of pain management is known as positive reinforcement. This means that desirable behaviour results in the receipt by the patient of something that promotes continuity of the behaviour – a reward. Usually it is something that is enjoyed, or gives pleasure to the individual. Negative reinforcement means relief as a result of the removal of something unpleasant or feared, and it results in what is known as escape/avoidance conditioning (e.g. resting reduces pain). This is important in the production and maintenance of chronic maladaptive behaviours and it is difficult to change.

When behaviour has been established it is influenced both by the consequences it brings and stimuli in the environment that become 'cues' to the appearance of the behaviour. For example, firm links are established between taking analgesics at certain times of day and not others because of the link between drug consumption and pain relief. A wide variety of different stimuli provoke, increase or maintain maladaptive pain behaviours; these are known as antecedent or discriminative stimuli. The use of operant-conditioning techniques will extinguish or greatly modify abnormal illness behaviour in patients with pain. However, because cognition plays an active part in the establishment of maladaptive behaviours, and their extinction, it was realized that exposure to operant conditioning alone was insufficient as a treatment. The development of cognitive theory, combined with aspects of behavioural theory, led to the development of cognitive/behavioural therapy. This now forms the basis of psychological treatment for many chronic pain states, as described in Chapter 18.

The psychological basis of disability

It is recognized that psychological factors have a marked influence on pain and disability and that their effects may be greater than biomedical factors with respect to the outcome of treatment for chronic pain. We now know that the most important psychological factors promoting the process of conversion from acute to chronic pain and disability include beliefs about, and attitudes towards, pain, coping strategies, emotional distress and pain behaviours.

It is necessary in the context of this section of the chapter to understand the difference between disability and handicap. The World Health Organization's definitions of the two states are given in Box 5.3. As a practical illustration of the differences,

---

Box 5.3

Definitions of disability and handicap

Definition of Disability, World Health Organization, 1980

'A disability is any restriction or lack (resulting from an impairment) of ability to perform an activity in the manner or within the range considered normal for a human being.'

Definition of Handicap, World Health Organization, 1980

'A handicap is a disadvantage for a given individual, resulting from an impairment or disability, that limits or prevents the fulfilment of a role that is normal (depending on age, sex, social and cultural factors) for that individual.'

consider two men who suffer major trauma of a leg that leaves its use permanently impaired. This represents a disability. If one individual is a professional footballer his career may be brought to an end by the disability, whereas a man of similar age in a sedentary job is able to continue working although he has the same disability. The level of handicap of the former, however, is much greater than that of the latter with respect to his capacity for work. People with a disability, by varying in the extent that they make an effort to overcome it, vary in their level of handicap.

Non-specific low back pain is a very common condition that tends to occur in acute episodes but may become chronic. Many of the studies of the process of transition from acute incapacity to long-term disability and chronic pain have been carried out on individuals suffering from this condition. In the mid 1980s work by Waddell, an orthopaedic surgeon, and Main, a clinical psychologist, revealed clearly for the first time that the disability associated with chronic non-specific low back pain is only partly explicable in terms of physical factors found at the time of examination. They discovered that psychological factors are almost as significant as contributors to the level of disability as those that are physical. They observed that psychological distress and pain behaviour are significant predictors of disability. Since that time a range of psychological factors, described earlier in this chapter, has been shown to play a major part in the development of disability. It can be concluded that negative thoughts, attitudes and emotions (emotional distress) are important factors in the transition from acute to chronic pain states. Therefore, those emotional changes must be regarded as important barriers to recovery, with obvious implications for rehabilitation.

Clinicians may unwittingly reinforce negative psychological factors, including fear and false beliefs about pain and its cause. They may worsen still further with the reduction or abolition of hope and by the generation of anger if treatments fail. The activities and attitudes of the family are important; those of the spouse or main carer are particularly significant, as these may reinforce negative thinking and emotion and increase disability by encouraging dependency, albeit unconsciously.

Self-assessment questions

5.1 Which of the following psychological theories are important in the management of chronic pain?

a. Psychoanalytic theory
b. Learning theory
c. Cognitive theory
d. Psychosomatic theory
e. Behavioural theory

5.2 Which of the following are important cognitive factors in pain states and the development of disability?

a. Attitudes and belief about pain
b. Neuroticism
c. Fear
d. Positive reinforcement
e. Expectancies about outcome
f. Beliefs about self-efficiency

5.3 What are the characteristics of the coping style of 'non-copers'?

a. Increased anxiety
b. Increased consumption of analgesic drugs
c. Social withdrawal
d. Reduced rest

5.4 What condition is characterized by the following?

a. Emotional exhaustion
b. Low sense of personal accomplishment despite increasing work
c. Collapse of self-esteem
d. Desire for success
e. Detachment from others

5.5 What is the difference between a disability and a handicap?

Clinical aspects of pain

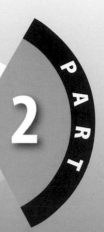

PART

2

Acute and chronic pain

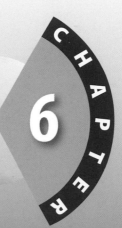

Chapter objectives

After studying this chapter you should be able to:

1 Differentiate between the biological and psychological characteristics of acute and chronic pain.

2 Describe the consequences of untreated or inadequately treated acute and chronic pain.

3 Describe the value of knowledge of the nature and anatomical distribution of acute pain in diagnosis.

4 Understand why diagnosis of the cause of chronic pain does not always enable curative treatment, and that management of pain and optimization of function then become the goals of treatment.

The characteristics of acute and chronic pain

Acute pain develops as a result of tissue damage caused by stimuli such as trauma, tumour or inflammation and muscle ischaemia. In certain instances, pain does not follow trauma, for example for a short period after major accidental trauma, or in battle immediately after wounding. There is a rare condition known as 'congenital indifference to pain' in which, as a result of certain neurotransmitter abnormalities, the individual does not feel pain at all and suffers major injuries as a result of burns, falls and other traumas, eventually dying at an early age. Acute pain has definite value to the sufferer because it draws attention to the underlying cause and it initiates behaviour that is designed to abolish pain as quickly as possible. The main emotions aroused by it are anxiety and, at times, fear. In contrast, pain that persists for more than 6 months is regarded as chronic and, by those who suffer it, such pain often comes to be regarded as 'useless': an experience from which there seems to be no escape and that does not have any benefits. Chronic pain provokes complex patterns of emotion and behaviour. The main emotions are low mood with the possibility of anxiety and fear, especially when new symptoms appear or treatments fail. Anger is also a feature of many chronic pain states, although not always identified by healthcare professionals.

Acute pain

Acute pain is common. The most common cause is trauma; this is the commonest cause of morbidity and mortality in people under the age of 24 years. In 1994 injury was listed first out of 29 conditions in the United States when ranked in terms of hospital days generated. Relatively little is known about the scale of painful injuries as a result of accidents, but figures for mortality indicate that the number of deaths in the world from trauma will increase from around five million in 1990 to about eight and a half million in 2020. The scale of acute pain due to injury alone can be imagined with these figures as a background.

Despite the high frequency with which people present to prehospital care and accident and emergency departments with painful injuries in the United Kingdom, the treatment of their pain is often poor. A UK government report in 2000 indicated that lack of personnel dedicated to pain relief was the prime cause. In contrast, acute pain teams have been estab-

Box 6.1

Effects of acute pain

- 50% of postsurgical patients, and those who suffer trauma, experience severe to intolerable pain.
- Poorly controlled postsurgical pain, and pain after trauma, is a risk factor for myocardial infarctions, pneumonia and deep venous thrombosis.
- Severe, acute and poorly controlled pain after surgery increases the risk of persistent pain in the longer term. Chronic pain after surgery and trauma is common and debilitating.

lished in hospital wards. They tend to concentrate their efforts on the relief of postoperative pain, and yet there is still inadequate provision of such services. Patients with acute pain from other causes, for example elderly patients with rib, vertebral and hip fractures, patients having dressing or pressure sore care and those with visceral pain such as pancreatitis, are often poorly managed.

Why should we want to abolish acute pain? The obvious answer is to relieve the suffering of patients. Furthermore, acute pain, if unchecked, has deleterious effects upon the ventilatory, cardiovascular, alimentary, urogenital and immune systems (Box 6.1). Relief of acute pain reduces morbidity and mortality and allows more rapid resumption of everyday activities that promote a more rapid general recovery. The potentially harmful effects of untreated, or inadequately treated, acute pain are well illustrated by considering its effect following upper abdominal surgery. Pain stimulates reflex 'muscle splinting' at the level of, and either side of, the site of an incision by causing spasm of abdominal and intercostal muscles. Untreated patients exhibit forced expiration against the muscle spasm and lung function is compromised (Fig. 6.1). This leads to areas of lung collapse, or atelectasis, and hypoxaemia that, coupled with the inability to cough and clear secretions because of pain, increases the chance of chest infection. Such changes occur more readily in smokers, obese patients, those with a history of chest disease and the elderly. The elderly in particular are susceptible to respiratory complications following abdominal or thoracic surgery because they have weaker muscles, are often poorly nourished and have a greater tendency to immobility. There is also a risk of pressure sores and

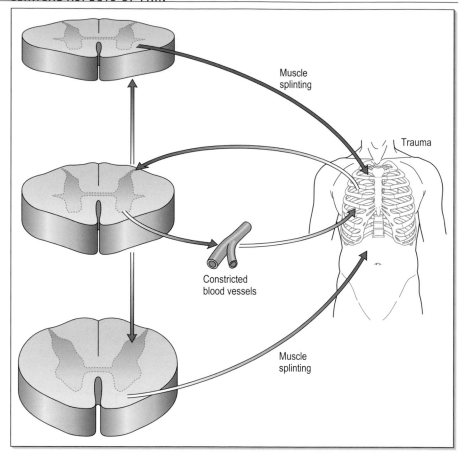

Fig 6.1 Some effects of postoperative pain on the chest and abdominal walls. Following the trauma of surgery there is pain, muscle spasm in the chest wall and increased sympathetic activity. Interneuronal activity spreads over several segments of the spinal cord (above and below the level of the stimulus). Neuronal activity results in widespread motor and autonomic activity. Muscle spasm is painful and reinforces the process. Reproduced from Cousins MJ & Phillips GD (eds). Acute Pain Management. Churchill Livingstone, 1986.

of thromboembolism if pain prevents patients from mobilizing after surgery.

Acute pain stimulates the sympathetic nervous system and the resulting tachycardia, vasoconstriction and hypertension may be dangerous for patients who have a history of myocardial ischaemia (angina or infarction) or vascular disease. Cardiac work and oxygen demand may outstrip supply leading to angina or infarction.

Problems with gastrointestinal function occur in the presence of unrelieved acute pain; for example nausea and vomiting may be a problem. Increased sympathetic activity results in increased gastric secretion but, as a result of a reduction in smooth muscle tone and activity, there is a reduction of gut motility and gastric stases results. These factors may also contribute to the occurrence of postoperative ileus (paralysis of the small bowel). In addition, opioid drugs commonly used in the treatment of acute pain reduce gastric motility and emptying causing emesis (vomiting) and slow bowel transit time. Therefore in some circumstances it is important to use analgesic techniques that avoid using large doses of opioid (e.g. regional anaesthetics or anti-inflammatory drugs). Increased sympathetic activity also affects the function of the bladder and may result in urinary retention by increasing bladder neck sphincter tone. Opioid drugs may compound this problem.

Acute pain may increase the stress response to surgery, and modulates the immunological response to trauma. There is conflicting evidence about the role of pain management in mitigating these effects. It is likely that different analgesic techniques and drugs have different effects on the neuroendocrine and immune systems. Further research is needed to clarify this potentially important area.

These illustrations show that there are very important reasons for ensuring that patients experience the least possible postoperative pain. (For methods of acute pain relief see Ch. 15.)

The role of acute pain in diagnosis

The site and nature of acute pain is often a key diagnostic sign and, in some cases, the only sign of an underlying abnormality. In acute trauma, pain usually occurs at the site of the injury, but not always. For example, damage to the spleen with the release of blood in the abdomen leads to stimulation of the under surface of the diaphragm that is supplied by the C3/4 segments of the spinal cord, and therefore gives rise to referred pain in the region of the left shoulder tip. In acute pancreatitis, in addition to severe upper abdominal pain, back pain is experienced in the distribution of the sixth to tenth thoracic dermatomes. The pain from myocardial infarction is felt in the chest but, in addition, also in the left arm and hand and possibly in the jaw because the distribution of pain is in the dermatomes associated with the first to fifth thoracic segments of the spinal cord that supply these areas. Several segments in the spinal cord are reached by nociceptive stimuli travelling along afferent nerves in association with sympathetic nerves from the viscera. The visceral afferent fibres are far less numerous than

Table 6.1 Surface sites of referred pain from viscera

Organ	Sites of local and referred pain	Cord levels
Spleen	Abdomen and shoulder tip (L)	C3/4
Mediastinum	Retrosternal, neck, abdomen, arm	C8–T5
Gallbladder/ common bile duct	Upper right quadrant abdomen, back – right scapula	T6–T10
Pancreas	Upper abdomen, back at level L1	T6–T10
Kidney/ureter (renal stone)	Loin to groin and penis/vulva	T10–L2
Myocardial infarction	Retrosternal, left arm/trunk	T1–T5

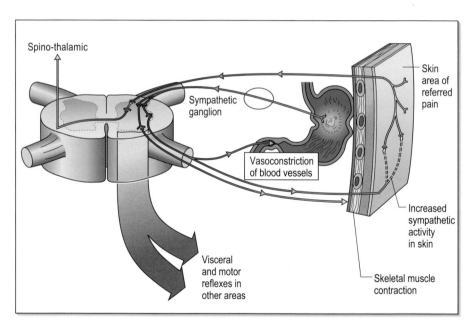

Fig 6.2 Pathways for referred pain from an abdominal organ. Visceral and somatic nociceptor neurons converge on the dorsal horn of the spinal cord. Pain is felt at the surface of the body in an area corresponding to the level of convergence. Note the effect also on the muscles of the body wall and visceral and vasomotor stimulation. Reproduced from Cousins MJ & Phillips GD (eds). Acute Pain Management. Churchill Livingstone, 1986.

those from the skin with which they converge in the dorsal horn of the spinal cord. Therefore, when there is visceral pathology, symptoms such as pain and hyperalgesia are experienced most clearly on the surface of the body (Table 6.1, Fig. 6.2). So it is important for the clinician to be able to distinguish

Table 6.2 Visceral pain compared with somatic pain

	Somatic	Visceral
Site	Well localized	Poorly localized
Radiation	May follow distribution of somatic nerve	Diffuse
Character	Sharp and definite	Dull and vague (may be colicky cramping, squeezing)
Relation to stimulus	Hurts at the site of the stimulus Associated with external causes	May be referred to another area Associated with internal causes
Time relations	Often constant though sometimes periodic	Often periodic and builds to peaks though sometimes constant
Associated symptoms	Nausea usually only with deep somatic pain owing to bone involvement	Often nausea, vomiting, sickening feeling

Adapted from Table 18.9, p. 298. Wall PD, Melzack R (eds) Textbook of pain, 3rd edn. Churchill Livingstone, Edinburgh. 1994. Reproduced with permission.

between pain that is somatic or visceral in origin. The main characteristics of the two types of pain are shown in Table 6.2. Table 6.3 identifies the spinal segments that receive the different visceral afferents.

Emotional consequences of acute pain

Anxiety and fear are generated by acute pain; this is important because they increase pain. Centres concerned with emotion in the brain link with, and increase the flow of information to, the descending inhibitory pathways from the brain; these modulate pain control within the spinal cord. Anxiety reinforces the sympathetic activity evoked by acute pain. Therefore, reduction of anxiety is a major requirement in the management of acute pain. Frequently the control of anxiety and fear, and of pain, is achieved by the administration of opioids. In addition, reduction of anxiety before surgical procedures by an explanation of

Table 6.3 Viscera and their segmental nociceptive nerve supply

Viscus	Spinal segments of visceral nociceptive afferents*
Heart	T1–T5
Lungs	T2–T4
Oesophagus	T5–T6
Stomach	T6–T10
Liver and gallbladder	T6–T10
Pancreas and spleen	T6–T10
Small intestine	T9–T10
Large intestine	T11–T12
Kidney and ureter	T10–L2
Adrenal glands	T8–L1
Testis, ovary	T10–T11
Urinary bladder	T11–L2
Prostate gland	T11–L1
Uterus	T10–L1

* These travel with sympathetic fibres and pass by way of sympathetic ganglia to the spinal cord. However, they are not sympathetic (afferent) fibres and are best referred to as visceral nociceptive afferents.

Note: Parasympathetic afferent fibres may be important in upper abdominal pain (vagal fibres, coeliac plexus).

Table 19.8, p. 297. From Textbook of pain. Wall PD, Melzack R (eds). 3rd edn. Churchill Livingstone, Edinburgh. 1994. Reproduced with permission.

the nature of the procedure with an emphasis upon its safety and the high likelihood of recovery significantly reduces post-operative anxiety, pain and analgesia requirements. The introduction of patient-controlled analgesia has given patients control over their pain management and, with that, reinforcement of self-efficacy. Knowing that they can control the dosage of analgesia may reduce their anxiety.

Chronic pain

Pain that persists beyond the point where it has value as an indicator of tissue damage is regarded as chronic. Although it can be argued that there cannot be any set time for this to happen, a current convention states that pain present for more than 6 months is chronic pain. However, people suffering from

Box 6.2

Characteristics of chronic pain

- Chronic pain is often regarded by the sufferer as 'useless' pain because it does not seem to serve any obvious purpose as a warning of danger.
- Chronic pain varies greatly in nature and intensity.
- Complaints of pain may be disproportionate to any underlying pathology.
- The most damaging effects of chronic pain are psychological and social.
- Psychological factors, anxiety, anger, and depression particularly, increase pain severity and reduce tolerance of it.
- Dependence on a variety of analgesic drugs is possible.

chronic pain may also often remain subject to episodes of acute pain, for example in cancer when the tumour has spread, or when a pathological fracture has occurred.

Chronic pain may, on the one hand, be the consequence of active and progressive diseases, for example cancer, rheumatoid arthritis or Crohn's disease of the bowel. On the other hand it may be the consequence of an acute disorder that has left residual tissue damage, as happens in postherpetic neuralgia and post-traumatic states. Chronic pain may occur as a consequence of degenerative changes in the joints of the limbs and spine.

Significance to the sufferers of the condition causing the pain, the coping strategies they adopt and the mood changes they experience all influence the severity and pattern of chronic pain (Box 6.2). Helping patients to cope by strengthening positive strategies and by giving them the belief that they will be able to control their pain are important aspects of chronic pain management (Ch. 16). With reference to the significance of the underlying condition, in many patients a diagnosis of cancer results in anxiety, fear and depression. Apart from dealing with physical aspects of disease, therefore, attention to emotional and spiritual needs is a major aspect of cancer pain management. In cancer there is the preoccupation with the possibility of death, but patients often have other significant concerns that include loss of their earning capacity and alterations in their family and social life, and other potential disruptive life-changes (Ch. 17).

The commonest cause of non-cancer chronic pain is low back pain and the emotions generated can vary significantly even within the same person. Usually they experience irritability and at times are bad tempered; they are often frustrated and angry. Periodic episodes of low mood or, at times, major depressive disorders occur especially in those who have a previous history of such disorders. Behaviour shown by patients with chronic pain varies. At one extreme are those who cope well, meaning that they make every effort to live their lives as normally as possible despite pain, and they show relatively little evidence of emotional disturbance. At the other extreme are those who retreat into chronic invalidism with a high level of dependency on others. This is often accompanied by frequent irritability, mood changes and possibly a depressive illness. A relatively common additional problem in patients with chronic pain is psychological or physical dependence on opioids and other analgesics. Generally such drugs have not been obtained on the street, but from doctors who, though well meaning, have not found an alternative way to provide pain management. The use of opioids in non-cancer pain is controversial. Many countries have produced recommendations about this issue, for example the British, Australian and American Pain Societies.

Physical accompaniments of chronic pain include poor sleep and tiredness, the possibility of weight loss, and side effects of medication. Illness itself may well produce tiredness and, rather than weight loss, some patients gain significant amounts of weight as a result of inactivity induced by the presence of chronic pain. Often patients supplement medically prescribed analgesia and, as a result, expose themselves to drug toxicity. This may occur when patients purchase paracetamol or anti-inflammatory drugs over the counter after the doctor has already prescribed the drug in another form.

Chronic pain and disability

Persistent acute pain becomes intermediate pain and, after 6 months, chronic pain. In the second stage, depression, frustration, anger and associated complex behavioural patterns emerge. These changes are related to the premorbid psychological characteristics of the patient and are influenced by physical and socioeconomic factors. Therefore, there is considerable interpatient variability in presentation. Research into the reasons for chronic low back pain disability has changed the treatment of this condition in the acute stage in recent years. At one time it was believed that long periods of bed rest were needed to overcome acute back pain. It has since been realized that, contrary to being beneficial, remaining in bed for more than 24 to 48 hours may well be counterproductive. In the absence of any signs of serious pathology or neurological localizing signs, patients are encouraged to mobilize as soon as possible and carry on their daily activities as normally as possible. Functional restoration is the main treatment goal in those with simple low back pain.

It is clear that psychological factors are important in the development of chronic pain from acute states. Chronic pain is associated with disability, work loss and claims for sickness benefits. Certain psychological factors in the acute pain state are strong predictors of the outcome of treatment. The presence of emotional distress, preoccupation with physical symptoms, anxiety, depression, negative beliefs about pain and poor coping strategies all predict a poor outcome and the development of chronic pain. There is some evidence that employment factors, such as poor job satisfaction, also have a role in ongoing disability. In the case of acute low back pain of less than 3 weeks' duration, the most significant predictor of disability at 1 year is the use of inappropriate coping strategies rather than the actual degree of physical impairment. These observations have led to a conclusion that psychosocial factors are better predictors of chronic low back pain and disability than clinical or physical signs and symptoms (see Box 6.2). A more detailed account of the development of disability is given in Chapter 5.

Self-assessment questions

Answer 'True' or 'False' to the following statements:

6.1 Acute pain is:

    a. Common

    b. Well managed in the community

    c. Well managed postoperatively

    d. Associated with respiratory, circulatory and gastro-intestinal complications after trauma or surgery if not controlled

    e. A source of anxiety and fear

6.2 Chronic pain is:

    a. Always a true indicator of underlying physical damage

    b. A cause of depression of mood

    c.   Sometimes a cause of drug dependence/addiction

    d.   A potential cause of long-term disability out of pro-portion to the underlying physical cause

6.3   Compared with somatic pain, visceral pain is:

    a.   Well located

    b.   May be referred to a distant area

    c.   Often periodic

Pain syndromes in the head, face and neck

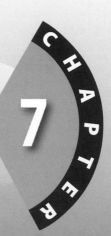

7

CHAPTER

Chapter objectives for Chapters 7 to 11

After studying these chapters you should be able to:

1 Describe the characteristic pains and associated symptoms in more common disorders of the head, face and neck, spine and limbs, thorax, abdomen and pelvis and the clinical presentation of certain generalized pain syndromes.

2 Describe the relationship between pain and a range of mental disorders.

3 Comment briefly on the overall management of pain and other symptoms in the disorders described (more detailed aspects of available management are given in Chapters 14–18).

Pain in the head and face

Headaches, and pains due to sinus or dental disease, are the commonest pain disorders of the head and facial region. Ocular causes for pain, in particular in acute infections and acute glaucoma, are important sources of pain in the head and face. Head and facial pain may be referred from the temporo-mandibular joints or the neck. Neuralgias involving one or other of the cranial nerves are uncommon. However, postherpetic neuralgia involving one of the divisions of the fifth cranial nerve and trigeminal neuralgia of the non-infective type are difficult problems to manage as they commonly affect older people. Head pain from primary or secondary malignancy is greatly feared by patients and their carers, but is relatively uncommon.

Headache

The epidemiological characteristics and classification of various forms of headache were described in Chapter 2.

Acute and chronic tension headache

Acute and, to a lesser extent, chronic tension headaches affect many people in the general population. The term 'tension' is applied to the consequences of emotional stress that gives rise to pain. There is a link between anxiety, depression and anger and increased tension in the scalp or neck muscles, although physiological evidence of such muscle tension is not always present. The characteristics of tension-type headache according to the most recent definition of The International Headache Society (2004) are given in Box 7.1.

The pain of tension headache may be described as dull and diffuse, as a band around the head or pressure on the head. It is not a throbbing pain and is not associated with nausea, vomiting, or photophobia. There may be, however, complaints of tenderness of the scalp and neck muscles.

The onset is usually gradual. Recurrent attacks occur with varying frequency and often the sufferer can relate them to a particular period of stress or tension.

Treatment of tension headache is that of the underlying emotional problem and help may be gained from relaxation, by using tricyclic antidepressants in small doses, or using biofeedback techniques. Of these options, removal of the causes of tension and the use of relaxation techniques are the most useful means of combating the attacks of pain.

Box 7.1

Diagnostic criteria for episodic tension-type headache

A At least 10 previous headache episodes fulfilling criteria B–D listed below.

B Headache lasting from 30 minutes to 7 days.

C At least two of the following pain characteristics:

    1   Pressing/tightening (non-pulsating) quality.

    2   Mild or moderate intensity.

    3   Bilateral location.

    4   No aggravation by walking, stairs, or similar routine physical activity.

D Both of the following:

    1   No nausea or vomiting (anorexia may occur).

    2   Photophobia and phonophobia are absent, or one but not the other is present.

International Headache Society 2004. From: The International Classification of Headache Disorders, 2edn. Cephalalgia, vol. 24, suppl 1, 2004. Reproduced with permission of Blackwell, Oxford.

In considering the diagnosis of tension headache, it must be distinguished from migraine. The crucial differences between the two are that, in the case of migraine sufferers only, there is often a family history of migraine; patients usually find that headache is made worse by physical activity and photophobia; visual disturbances and other localizing signs can occur. Anorexia is common, as is nausea, and to a lesser extent vomiting. Other possible causes of headache include eye, ear, or sinus conditions, pain arising from pathology in the cervical spine, intracerebral lesions and chronic abuse of analgesics. Formal psychiatric disorders can cause headache and, most commonly, a major depressive episode.

Migraine with aura (see also Ch. 2)

The diagnostic criteria for migraine, defined by the International Headache Society in 2004, are summarized in Box 7.2. The throbbing headache of this condition is often preceded by a prodromal state when the sufferer can experience an aura that is usually visual and can take various forms. It may be experienced as blurring, or flickering, the presence of a scotoma, (a patch of lost vision) or fortification spectra, which

Box 7.2

Diagnostic criteria for migraine without and with aura

A At least five attacks fulfilling B–D.

B Headache attacks lasting 4–72 hours.

C Headache has at least two of the following characteristics:

　　1 Unilateral location.

　　2 Pulsating quality.

　　3 Moderate or severe intensity (inhibits or prohibits daily activities).

　　4 Aggravation by walking, stairs, or similar routine physical activity.

D During headache at least one of the following:

　　1 Nausea and/or vomiting.

　　2 Photophobia and/or phonophobia.

E For 'Headache with aura' add:

　　1 Aura.

International Headache Society 2004. From: The International Classification of Headache Disorders, 2edn. Cephalalgia, vol. 24, suppl 1, 2004. Reproduced with permission of Blackwell Publishing, Oxford.

are zig-zag lines (Fig. 7.1). In addition, there may be a mood change in the direction of euphoria, food cravings, or weight gain because of water retention. The prodromal phase may last for up to a day before the headache begins, but lasts usually for no more than half an hour to an hour. The pain of migraine varies in severity, it is typically unilateral, although it may be bilateral, and it is throbbing in nature and associated with nausea, photophobia and perhaps vomiting. The duration of pain varies, but usually it lasts for 4 to 72 hours. A marked diuresis may follow the period of headache. Attacks of migraine mostly begin in adolescence or early adult life, but they are reduced significantly in pregnancy and may diminish with increasing age. A number of factors may be associated with the onset of migraine and they vary from person to person. They include foods rich in tyramine including chocolate, cheese, marmite and bananas. In some cases the precipitant is red wine, or a fortified wine such as sherry or brandy. Psychological factors may precipitate episodes of migraine and they include the effects of prolonged stress. Migraine tends to develop at the end of a stressful period, for example at weekends, or

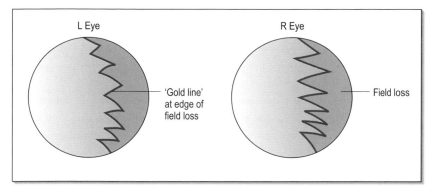

Fig 7.1 Right visual field loss during an acute episode of migraine with aura.

during the first few days of a holiday. It may occur during episodes of anxiety or depression in those susceptible to it.

Although neurological complications may develop because of migraine, they are very uncommon. They include hemianopia, the possibility of a mild hemiparesis (hemiplegic migraine), sensory changes in the hand or face, and dysphasia. Migraine may be treated with prophylactic drugs such as pizotifen or aspirin. Many sufferers are able to abort acute attacks of migraine with simple analgesics (paracetamol) alone, if combined with an antiemetic, or with a non-steroidal anti-inflammatory preparation. Others require potent substances that block the activity of serotonin and in particular the triptans. An acute attack of migraine may be treated effectively with metoclopramide, which though often given to relieve nausea is effective in reducing headache when given parenterally. Overuse of drugs may transform episodes of migraine into more frequent and continuous attacks.

Common migraine (migraine without aura)

Common migraine has all the features of classical migraine other than the development of an aura before the onset of an attack. Otherwise, the familial factors and the range of precipitants is much the same, as is treatment.

Cluster headache, short-lasting unilateral neuralgic form headache (SUNCT syndrome)

Cluster headaches, which are more common in men than women, consist of severe episodic attacks of pain that occur unilaterally in and around the eye spreading to the frontal and temporal regions. Cluster headaches occur in groups at intervals varying from weeks to months, hence the use of the term 'cluster'. The pain is associated with lacrimation, conjunctival infection, nasal stuffiness, photophobia and at times nausea. In some cases, when the symptoms are severe, irregularities of heart rhythm occur.

The causative factors are similar to those described for migraine and it is known that the consumption of alcohol during the course of a bout of headaches will precipitate an attack almost immediately, and any existing headache will become much more severe. The treatment for cluster headaches is the same as for the migraines.

Post-traumatic headache

Following an injury to the head, often a minor one, a non-specific generalized aching pain develops. In some cases, the pain is quite severe and is associated with photophobia, nausea and possibly vomiting. Post-traumatic headache is associated with variability of the mood, and in particular with irritability. The sufferer complains of poor concentration and memory, suggesting mild cerebral dysfunction, and there may be complaints of dizziness (the whole complex of symptoms constitutes the 'postconcussional syndrome'). The condition may last for weeks to months and in the latter case further psychological problems may develop, particularly feelings of depression and severe memory loss. They are not caused by brain injury but are secondary psychological consequences of the minor injury. In all cases a full clinical examination is required, including a radiological examination of the skull for evidence of fractures and, if necessary, MRI scanning for evidence of structural damage within the skull.

If dizziness and vertigo develop at the time of the injury then a disturbance of the organ of balance should be suspected. In most cases, these symptoms disappear within 12 months. Less common causes of headache are those related to pathological changes within the skull, including intracranial tumour, acute and subacute subdural haematomas.

Facial pain

Toothache and sinus pain

Toothache is a very common cause of oral pain. Three possibilities need to be considered, which are:

- Dental caries, a tooth fracture or cracked enamel, or a lost tooth filling.

- Inflammation of the dental pulp – pulpitis. This condition is a complication of deeply invading dental caries that has extended into the pulp cavity. When the condition is mild, pain is experienced only with direct stimulation of the tooth, but with its progression a constant pain develops which is increased by the application of heat or cold. If untreated the dental pulp will die and a root abscess may form.

- Periapical periodontitis or a root abscess, which may be secondary to pulpitis. This condition presents as a constant throbbing pain in the gums and face with swelling of the latter and varying in intensity. It may appear to arise from more than one tooth. Stimulation of the teeth with percussion, heat or cold should identify the site of the infection.

The treatment of these conditions is by dental surgery.

Maxillary sinusitis

This condition presents as a dull aching pain in the region of the frontal or maxillary sinuses and it is associated with a sense of fullness and tenderness of the overlying skin that may be flushed and, in the case of the cheek, slightly swollen. Pain extends into the teeth of the upper jaw in a maxillary infection and bending forwards increases the pain. The cause of the pain is an infection associated with blocking of the outlet of the sinus by infected material and swelling of the mucosa, or occasionally by tumour. It may also be dental in origin. Radiological examination of the sinus reveals that the mucosa is thickened and that there is fluid within the sinus cavity.

Early treatment is by the use of antibiotics, but surgical intervention is needed if the condition is severe, if it involves a carious tooth, or if it is chronic and sinus drainage is needed.

Temporomandibular joint pain (temporomandibular pain and dysfunction syndrome)

This syndrome has a number of features including tenderness of the muscles of mastication in the temporal region, around the ear and at the angle of the jaw. Pain may be experienced in the sternomastoid muscles. It is usually unilateral, dull and aching in nature and is associated with brief episodes of severe pain when the sufferer chews food or yawns. Often the movements of jaw are restricted with limited mouth opening (trismus) and the sufferer may report clicking or popping sounds from the region of the joint. The pain is often most severe on wakening and especially if there has been clenching of the teeth during sleep (bruxism). Paradoxically the pain seldom wakens the individual. It results sometimes from malocclusion of the teeth or because of bruxism (grinding of the teeth and especially during sleep), in which case the pain is usually bilateral. Bruxism is generally a sign of emotional tension.

A radiological examination of the joint may not reveal any evidence of abnormality, although on occasions there are signs of osteoarthritis or rheumatoid arthritis. Arthrography may reveal a displacement of the disc within the joint to a variable extent and a similar finding may be present on an MRI scan. The significance of the displacement of the disc within the joint is uncertain unless it is the result of definite trauma.

The condition tends to pursue a fluctuating course and treatment involves use of night splints. The value of surgical treatment is debated and a matter for specialist consideration.

Psychological factors, and in particular those associated with stress and anxiety, are often present in patients with the syndrome and resolution of these issues is regarded by many as an important aspect of treatment of the condition.

Facial pain associated with psychological problems

Apart from pain arising from the temporomandibular joint(s), pain in the face may develop in the course of a psychiatric disorder and, in particular, in those suffering from a major depressive episode. A physical examination and appropriate investigations must be performed when there is a physical basis for the complaint of dull, aching pain that occurs at any site on the face, or at times as dental pain. The sufferer is frequently a middle-aged woman and careful questioning may reveal evidence of a depressive disorder rather than a physical cause. Such pain is often termed atypical facial pain, and in terms of the biopsychosocial model (see Ch. 5) it is typical of an emotional problem. Failure to check for evidence of an emotional disorder leads to unnecessary investigations, perhaps unnecessary treatments of a surgical nature, and a persistence of the disorder.

Neuralgias affecting the face

The main sensory nerves to the face are distributed through the three divisions of the trigeminal nerve. Structures supplied by the ninth and twelfth cranial nerves include the tongue, palate, pharynx and larynx and certain neck muscles. The cutaneous supply of the scalp and neck is largely via the cervical nerves. Any of the nerves in this group may be the site of neu-ralgic pain.

*Trigeminal neuralgia
(tic douloureux)*

Middle-aged and older people experience this condition as a recurrent severe, and at times agonizing, unilateral brief stabbing pain that lasts only seconds in one or more divisions of the trigeminal nerve. Often it is triggered by light stimulation such as washing or shaving. The pain shows variable periodicity with pain-free intervals that may last for weeks or months. Sensory testing of the facial skin and cornea may not reveal any evidence of abnormality other than triggering of the pain by light touch.

The cause of trigeminal neuralgia in most cases is a lesion compressing the trigeminal nerve at its exit from the brain-stem, most often a small artery that can be seen on MR–angi-ography. In some cases it occurs in multiple sclerosis and then usually in early adult life.

The standard treatment for trigeminal neuralgia, and other neuralgias of the head and face, is based upon the use of anti-convulsant drugs (e.g. carbamazepine or gabapentin). Antide-pressant drugs such as amitriptyline and venlafaxine have been used as coanalgesics. Baclofen has been used with variable results. Definitive surgical treatment involves either microvas-cular decompression of the trigeminal root if the patient is fit enough, or section of the fibres of the appropriate division of the nerve. Patients in a poor state of health may benefit from a radiofrequency lesion or glycerol injection of the trigeminal ganglion.

*Acute herpes zoster
(shingles)*

This disorder occurs in adults of either sex, chiefly in middle to old age, although occasionally it may occur in younger patients and in those with immune suppression (e.g. from chemotherapy). The most common sites are the trunk and in the elderly the facial skin supplied by one of the divisions of the trigeminal nerve; the cornea may be involved. The condition begins with the onset of a severe burning and tingling pain to which is added occasional lancinating pains. They precede the onset of the herpetic eruption of vesicles by 1 or 2 days. Often the pain disappears only to reappear after the skin eruption has subsided. It may persist for only a few days, or last for many months. Recovery occurs more readily in younger people and in the elderly it may unfortunately become a chronic condition. Treatment in the acute stage, and

Fig 7.2 Scarring in the first and second divisions of the left trigeminal nerve caused by Herpes Zoster virus.

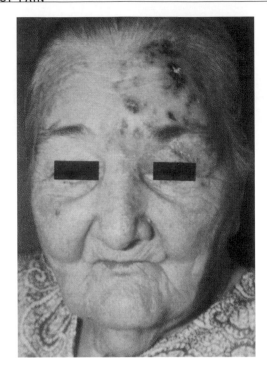

when the rash appears, is by systemic use of antiviral agents (e.g. Zovirax).

Postherpetic neuralgia (PHN)

Chronic pain can develop following herpes zoster infection affecting any dermatome and is due to central and peripheral nerve damage. One or more divisions of the trigeminal nerve can be involved (Fig. 7.2); the eye including the cornea can be affected. Herpes infections may involve the seventh cranial nerve, giving rise to severe lancinating pain in the distribution of the nerve, especially with talking, swallowing, coughing and yawning. Neuralgia of the ninth, or glossopharyngeal, nerve gives rise to stabbing pain in the ear and tonsillar region caused by swallowing, coughing and yawning. PHN is uncommon in young people, unless they are immune compromised. It is more frequent in the elderly and tends to affect men more often than women. PHN pain can be classified according to its quality; this probably reflects the different effects of the virus on different parts of the nervous system. The pain is severe, burning and constant. It is associated with an itching and crawling sensation in the skin and, at times, has a sharp stabbing component. It may occur spontaneously or be precipitated by light touch. The pain varies in severity and, although it may last for some years, tends to diminish with time. The chronicity and intensity of the pain are such that it may cause irritability and a major depressive disorder that, at times, results in suicide.

At the site of the pain the skin is scarred by infection and there may be loss of pigmentation. Examination often reveals hypoaesthesia and hypoalgesia; but allodynia and hyperpathia may occur.

Treatment of PHN is usually by a combination of simple analgesics and adjuvants such as anticonvulsant or antidepressant drugs, or both, for the control of both pain and mood. Opioids are helpful in the management of PHN, but side effects may be a problem and these need to be managed carefully, especially in elderly patients. Local application of capsaicin or a lidocaine patch may be useful, but not near the eye or genitalia. Local treatment with sympathetic blockade is controversial and often helpful only if performed early. TENS and acupuncture have been used; the evidence for success with these therapies is poor, but they are relatively non-invasive. Surgery and nerve ablation are usually useless and may actually increase pain.

Suboccipital and cervical disorders giving rise to pain

Cervicogenic headache (occipital neuralgia)

A relatively common form of neuralgia arises from structures in the neck, perhaps secondarily to a hyperextension or whiplash type injury occurring in a motor vehicle accident when the subject's car is struck from the rear. Moderate to severe deep aching pain occurs in the suboccipital region and, at times, there is a stabbing element. Usually it is located unilaterally and may radiate to the vertex, fronto-orbital region, or even the face. The pain is often associated with tenderness of the cervical muscles. Clinical examination may reveal diminished sensation in the dermatome of the second cervical nerve, and tenderness over the course of the greater occipital nerve as it travels upwards over the occiput. The course of the condition is chronic with periods of freedom and intermittent episodes of pain.

Other causes of pain of this type that should be considered include tumours in the higher cervical region, or the posterior fossa of the skull, and a herniated cervical disc, but all are uncommon.

Treatment of the pain is generally with analgesic drugs and temporary relief may be gained by blocking the greater occipital nerve, or the second cervical nerve with a local anaesthetic agent with or without steroid. Acupuncture can be effective for this condition. Peripheral nerve stimulation using an implanted electrode and pulse generator has been successful in treating occipital neuralgia.

Glaucoma

Glaucoma is a disorder of the eye in which a sudden, or gradual increase in intraocular pressure results in damage to the sight with loss of vision if untreated. When intraocular pressure increases suddenly, extremely severe eye pain develops and vision is lost rapidly without urgent treatment. Acute glaucoma develops when the pupil dilates and drainage of fluid from the anterior chamber of the eye is obstructed. It is more common in 'long-sighted' people and can be caused by low lighting levels, or certain medications (e.g. tricyclic drugs). Less often the cause may be direct trauma to the eye and inflammation of the iris (iritis), or diabetes. The onset of the condition is sudden and symptoms usually occur in one eye only. Initially there is pain in the eye and head with slight visual loss. The subject describes seeing haloes around bright lights. Within a few hours, the pain becomes severe and there is a rapid loss of vision. The eye becomes red, it waters, the eyelid swells and the pupil dilates and becomes unresponsive to light. The iris takes on a cloudy appearance. In association with the local symptoms the sufferer experiences nausea and may vomit. Early treatment of acute glaucoma is essential if sight is to be preserved. It should be noted that attacks of acute glaucoma might recur. The intraocular pressure may be reduced by the oral administration of a carbonic anhydrase inhibitor but, given that the patient may be experiencing nausea and have vomited, the direct use in the eye of the cholinergic antagonist pilocarpine may be needed. This drug causes constriction of the ciliary muscle and that helps to open the drainage channels in the trabecular mesh between the iridocorneal junction and the Canal of Schlemm. Once control has been gained, the production of aqueous humour in the anterior chamber of the eye may be reduced by using beta-blocker drugs that produce minimal local adverse effects. However, drainage of the drops via the lacrimal duct and their absorption from the nasal mucosa into the general circulation can produce a reduction of blood pressure and slowing of the heart rate. Therefore, a cardioselective agent (e.g. betaxolol) is to be preferred to non-selective agents in the elderly and patients with heart disease or a history of bronchial asthma. The condition should be reviewed as a matter of urgency by an ophthalmic surgeon who may conclude that a surgical procedure is required to improve the drainage of the aqueous fluid.

Chronic glaucoma, which is the commoner form, is an insidious and slowly developing disorder that results in a gradual and painless loss of vision if it is undetected. Chronic glaucoma is generally manifest after the age of 35 years, and tends to occur in certain families. For that reason the close relatives of an individual found to have chronic glaucoma as a random event should be examined for evidence of further family involvement. In order to detect the condition in the general population it is recommended that every person over the age of 40 should undergo periodic eye tests involving simple measurements of intraocular pressure.

The treatment of chronic glaucoma may involve the use of a beta blocker to reduce production of fluid in the anterior chamber, the use of a carbonic anhydrase inhibitor that has a similar effect, or non-steroidal anti-inflammatory drugs given as local drops to both eyes.

Self-assessment questions

7.1 Which of the following symptoms are experienced in common migraine?

    a. Headache
    b. Photophobia
    c. Visual aura
    d. Onset related to specific foods or drinks
    e. Nausea and vomiting

7.2 Which of the following symptoms occur in acute glaucoma?

    a. Headache
    b. Nausea and vomiting
    c. Fortification spectra
    d. Pain in the eye
    e. Sight loss

7.3 Which two of the following are *not* used in the treatment of trigeminal neuralgia?

    a. Carbamazepine
    b. Paracetamol
    c. Baclofen
    d. Gabapentin
    e. Morphine sulphate

7.4 What do the following symptoms – headache, photophobia, nausea, irritability and late onset of depression indicate?

a. Cluster headache

b. Simple glaucoma

c. Post-traumatic syndrome

d. Intracranial tumour

Spinal and radicular pain

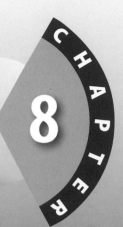

CHAPTER

8

Chapter objectives for Chapters 7 to 11

After studying these chapters you should be able to:

1 Describe the characteristic pains and associated symptoms in more common disorders of the head, face and neck, spine and limbs, thorax, abdomen and pelvis and the clinical presentation of certain generalized pain syndromes.

2 Describe the relationship between pain and a range of mental disorders.

3 Comment briefly on the overall management of pain and other symptoms in the disorders described (more detailed aspects of available management are given in Chs 14–18).

Radicular pain

Radicular pain is experienced as the result of ectopic stimulation of the nerve at some point along its course, for example by mechanical deformation (as in the case of a prolapsed intervertebral lumbar disc), inflammation or ischaemia, and not as a result of the stimulation of the peripheral nerve endings. As a result, radicular pain differs from referred pain in terms of its mode of origin. Referred pain is felt as a deep and rather diffuse aching sensation without a cutaneous element, whereas radicular pain is lancinating, stabbing or shooting, and is accompanied by sensory changes such as tingling or numbness. In addition, there may be a background dull ache. The area of the pain is well defined and often located within a specific dermatome or dermatomes. Therefore, it is felt both at the level of the skin and more deeply (Fig. 8.1).

Radiculopathy

Whereas radicular pain is due to ectopic stimulation of a peripheral nerve, a radiculopathy is a condition in which there is a conduction block of a nerve or its roots with clinically detectable loss of sensory or motor function. In other words, the causative lesion blocks conduction directly by mechanical compression, or indirectly by affecting the blood supply or nutrition of the nerve. The conduction block may be demonstrated electrophysiologically in nerve conduction studies, for example in the 'carpal tunnel syndrome'. It may occur either in isolation, with radicular pain, referred pain, or direct spinal pain.

Spinal and radicular syndromes of the cervical region

Radicular pain, that is pain originating from a spinal nerve, may be due to one of several categories of disorder that include the consequences of trauma, for example, vertebral fractures (Fig. 8.2), disc protrusions and nerve compressions, a direct nerve injury, or the presence of an infection (tuberculosis), at some point on the pathway of the nerve. It may be due to the pressure of a tumour, which could be benign or malignant, including tumours of the nerves themselves. Other causes include degenerative changes in bone, such as osteoarthritis, rheumatoid arthritis and, less commonly, ankylosing spondylitis, or as the result of a congenital abnormality of the vertebra, for example in congenital spinal scoliosis.

Fig 8.1 Anterior and posterior dermatomes

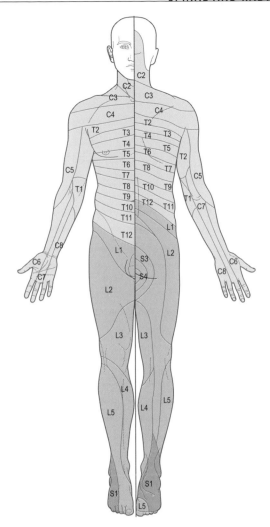

Commoner causes of cervical radicular pain

Acute cervical sprain (an acceleration–deceleration injury often termed 'whiplash injury')
Neck pain affects more than one in 10 of adults. Acute cervical sprain occurs when there is a jerking injury of the neck with hyperextension followed by flexion with or without a rotational element. Such injuries occur classically in rear end motor vehicle collisions or 'shunting' accidents. During the first 24 hours following the accident, the affected individual develops an aching pain in the neck muscles often radiating into the trapezius muscles on one or both sides. Next, muscle spasm develops in many cases leading to total inability to move the head in any direction. Examination at that point may well reveal evidence of 'trigger points', which are areas of acute tenderness in the muscles of the neck and shoulders. The pain may extend upwards over the occipital region. The precise

Fig 8.2 A crush fracture at L1.

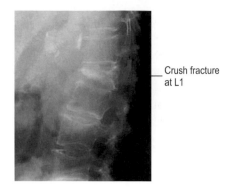

Crush fracture at L1

reason for the onset of pain is uncertain, but is believed to be strain of muscles and ligaments surrounding the joints of the neck, and in particular the facet joints, at the site of the injury. Evidence of bony injury on radiological examination is usually absent, although there may be pre-existing arthritic changes, often non-symptomatic, that could have been aggravated by the injury. Radiological examination may also reveal loss of the usual curvature of the cervical spine indicating the presence of muscle spasm. More detailed information is obtained by the use of MRI. Apart from pain in the neck and head the sufferers may experience it in one or both arms and hands. Other symptoms that sometimes accompany pain include dizziness, tinnitus, blurring of vision, disturbances of sleep, and depression of mood may be a psychological reaction in more severe cases. The symptoms, and particularly pain, may last for 1 to 2 years and become chronic in approximately 10% of those afflicted.

Treatment of the condition is primarily by means of analgesics, non-steroidal anti-inflammatory drugs and the early use of muscle relaxants. Early physiotherapy to relieve muscle spasm and to improve movement is an essential feature of treatment. The use of a cervical support collar, other than for a very brief period of time, is not recommended.

Chronic neck pain The most common cause of chronic neck pain is degenerative changes in the cervical spine (cervical spondylosis), which is present in 75% of the population over the age of 50 years. Despite the frequency with which this condition occurs, most who have it are free from pain, but experience limitations of movements of the neck and may describe a grating sensation when rotating the head. A clear correlation between the extent of degenerative changes seen on radiological examination and the presence of pain is poor. Changes in the cervical spine with age, as with those that occur in both the thoracic and lumbar regions, include degenerative changes in the fibrocartilagenous discs, which shrink and narrow, the development of bony protrusions or osteophytes at the margins of the vertebrae, thickening of joint ligaments and possibly narrowing of the foramina through which spinal nerves leave the spinal canal. Degenerative changes of facet joints in the vertebrae occur and cervical pain may arise from them.

The pain of cervical spondylosis is experienced as a dull ache, rather like toothache, which occurs throughout the cervical region, although more towards the lower half with episodes of more severe pain, at times perhaps associated with muscle spasm. Compression of spinal nerve roots as a result of the processes described will lead to dull aching pains extending from the neck into the arms and hands; in other words a cervical radiculopathy develops. The most severe changes in cervical spondylosis tend to occur at the junctions of the fifth and sixth and the sixth and seventh vertebrae where spinal movements are greatest (with the exception of the level 1/2). Pain and changes in sensation occur in the distribution of the cervical nerves at that level and often unilaterally. The natural history of cervical spondylosis with an associated radiculopathy is that it is present intermittently with bouts of freedom lasting for a period of days to many weeks.

Rarely, a cervical disc prolapse occurs leading to cervical radiculopathy with severe pain, associated muscle wasting and weakness and dermatomal sensory changes in keeping with the affected nerve(s) (Box 8.1).

The basis of treatment for intermittent cervical pain and the radiculopathy of cervical spondylosis is the use of simple analgesics, for example paracetamol and of non-steroidal anti-inflammatory drugs. Immobilization of the neck at times of acute attacks of pain is helpful. In intractable cases, injection of cervical facet joints, or their denervation, may bring relief. Surgical intervention for nerve root compression is indicated only when there is clear evidence, via clinical examination and an MRI scan, of a cervical disc prolapse that has failed to respond to conservative management, or where a nerve root is compressed by osteophytes that may be removed.

Spinal and radicular pains of the thoracic region

Spinal and radicular pain originating from the thoracic spine may be due to an injury, with or without a fracture, infection of a vertebra or adjacent structures, and the presence of

Box 8.1

Typical findings in cervical root compression producing radicular pain or a radiculopathy

C5 root compression (C4–C5 disc)

- Pain – neck, shoulder, medial scapula, anterior chest, lateral aspect of upper arm
- Numbness – sometimes lateral upper arm or area over deltoid
- Weakness – deltoid, supraspinatus, infraspinatus, biceps, brachioradialis
- Hyporeflexia – biceps, brachioradialis reflexes

C6 root compression (C5–C6 disc)

- Pain – neck, shoulder, medial scapula, anterior chest, lateral aspect of upper arm, dorsal aspect of forearm
- Numbness – thumb and index finger (sometimes absent)
- Weakness – biceps (mild to moderate), extensor carpi radialis
- Hyporeflexia – biceps reflex

C7 root compression (C6–C7 disc)

- Pain – same as in C6 root compression
- Numbness – index and middle fingers (sometimes absent)
- Weakness – triceps
- Hyporeflexia – triceps reflex

C8 root compression (C7–T1 disc)

- Pain – neck, medial scapula, anterior chest, medial aspect of arm and forearm
- Numbness – fourth and fifth fingers, occasionally middle finger
- Weakness – triceps, all extensors of wrist and fingers except extensor carpi radialis; all flexors of wrist and fingers except flexor carpi radialis and palmaris longus, all intrinsic hand muscles
- Hyporeflexia – triceps reflex

T1 root compression (T1–T2 disc)

- Pain – same as in C8 root compression
- Numbness – ulnar aspect of forearm (usually subjective)
- Weakness – only intrinsic muscles of hand
- Hyporeflexia – none
- Miscellaneous – Horner's syndrome

malignant tumours either primary or secondary; of the two, the latter is most common – often from breast, lung or prostate. Pain may originate from degenerative changes, as for example in the presence of osteoarthritis, osteoporosis, rheumatoid arthritis and ankylosing spondylitis. Certain congenital conditions give rise to spinal pain and, in particular, congenital scoliosis. Pain due to a prolapsed intervertebral disc in the thoracic region is a rarity. Pain arising from osteoporosis of the thoracic spine is described in Chapter 10.

Acute mechanical back pain in the thoracic region

Pain results usually from acute minor trauma and presents as a deep aching pain with more severe pain above and below the site of the injury if muscle spasm occurs, as is commonly the case. There is limitation of movement and local tenderness with recovery in a matter of days to 4–6 weeks and treatment should be with simple analgesics, perhaps non-steroidal anti-inflammatory drugs, and the avoidance of movements that cause pain. Some limitation in activity may be necessary but that is not always the case. Simple backache of a more chronic type may be the result of bad posture, be associated with obesity, or be a consequence of chronic emotional stress.

In adolescents and young adults, complaints of persistent backache may be the result of congenital abnormalities of the spine, for example kyphoscoliosis, or the onset of the rare condition of ankylosing spondylitis. Later in life, and in the middle-aged or older generations, degenerative changes give rise to chronic back pain, although this is experienced most often in the lumbar and cervical regions.

Ankylosing spondylitis

This condition is an inflammatory arthritic disorder that is uncommon and affects men more often than women. It makes its appearance in early adult life, that is before 40 years, and presents initially with complaints of low back pain and marked stiffness of the back on wakening that is eased by exercise. The onset is slow and starts in the region of the sacroiliac joints. It progresses gradually involving other joints as it ascends the spine. The extent of progression varies and, in some cases when the disability is mild, halts at an early stage. In contrast, in severe cases where the whole spine is involved it becomes completely ossified, leaving the sufferer bent like a bow and unable to look ahead because of the extreme degree of spinal flexion.

Fig 8.3 Ankylosing spondylitis of the cervical spine.

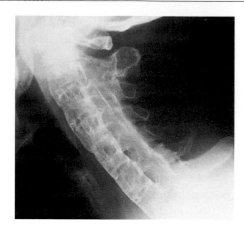

There may be a family history of the condition and associated disorders include iritis, colitis, urethritis and skin rashes, together with some involvement of peripheral joints. Radiological examination reveals sclerosis in the joints, and especially of those in the sacroiliac region, together with a typical change in the vertebrae leading to what is described as a 'bamboo spine' (Fig. 8.3).

Spinal and radicular pain in the lumbosacral and coccygeal regions

Acute mechanical low back pain

Low back pain is experienced by approximately 85% of adults by the age of 50. In 90% of those afflicted it is self-limiting and disappears within 2–4 weeks of onset; only 15–20% seek medical care, yet this is one of the most common conditions presenting to general practitioners. As with thoracic pain, though far more common, acute pain in the lumbosacral region is felt locally, but at times it radiates into the lower limbs. It is not associated with nerve root involvement or sphincter disturbance. At first there is often spasm of the lumbar muscles with local tenderness, or 'trigger points'. At times, muscle pain due to spasm may extend as high as the base of the skull.

The facet joints may be important in the generation of pain. Their anatomical position is shown in Figure 8.4. The synovial joints and their capsules are richly innervated by the posterior primary rami of spinal nerves. Injury, or degenerative changes in the joints, typically results in low back pain referred via the posterior primary rami of spinal nerves to the back and posterior thigh, and also via the lumbar anterior primary rami to the

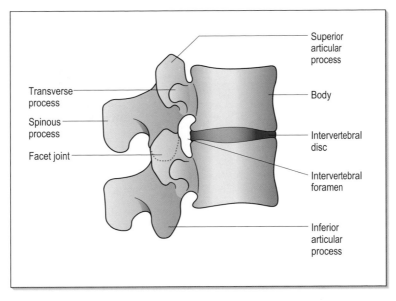

Superior
articular
process

Transverse
process

Body

Spinous
process

Facet joint

Intervertebral
disc

Intervertebral
foramen

Inferior
articular
process

Fig 8.4 Articulate vertebrae showing the position of a facet joint
(lateral view). Reproduced from Stannard CF & Booth S. Churchill's
Pocketbook of Pain 2 edn, Churchill Livingstone 2004.

lower abdomen, groin and thigh. Most often the pain is experienced in the region of the sacroiliac joints, buttocks and thighs.
The joints may be damaged by trauma, especially if degenerative processes are present. The mechanical load on the joints
increases after the removal of a prolapsed intervertebral disc
and they are subject to degenerative changes in rheumatoid
arthritis and osteoarthritis. A previously symptom-free joint
may give rise to pain after a sudden extension or twisting
injury of the lumbar spine, which unmasks a degenerative
condition. Often there is stiffness of the back on rising and on
examination, pain is experienced as a result of lumbar extension and pressure over the joint. In contrast, straight leg raising
and limb reflexes are normal. Often there is little correlation
between radiographic evidence of degeneration and low back
pain.

Between each vertebra lies an intervertebral disc, which is
an ovoid gelatinous mass, the nucleus pulposus, surrounded
by a strong annular ligament of fibrocartilage (Fig. 8.5). The
anterior and posterior longitudinal ligaments of the spine are
attached to the disc margins. Degenerative changes in the
annular ligament predispose it to rupture and when that
happens a fragment of the nucleus pulposus of variable size
is extruded posteriorly into the spinal canal (a disc prolapse,
Fig. 8.6). This results in compression and, more importantly,

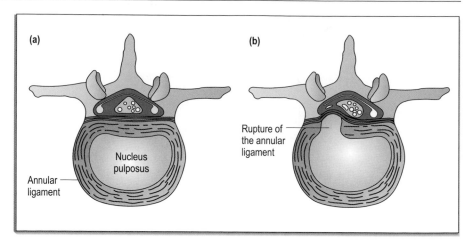

Fig 8.5 Anatomy of (a) a normal invertebral disc and (b) a disc prolapse.

Fig 8.6 MRI scan of an L5–S1. Prolapsed intervertebral disc, lumbo–sacral disc protrusion.

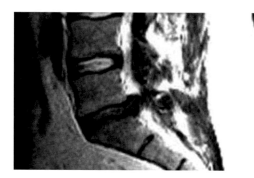

chemical irritation and inflammation of one or more spinal nerve roots in the intervertebral foramina. At the time of rupture of the annulus the patient may experience the sensation of popping in the lower back and immediately, although not always, severe low back pain develops. The inflammation and nerve root compression pain radiates into one or other leg except when the protrusion is central and then it is felt bilaterally. In association with nerve root compression, sensory diminution, or tingling and numbness, may develop in the appropriate dermatomes, usually of the L4/L5 and L5/S1 levels (Box 8.2 and Fig. 8.7).

Muscle weakness and wasting may occur too and the patient has a lumbar radiculopathy. Pain from a prolapsed disc is increased by straining, for example by coughing, bending, or defaecation.

The prolapse of a lumbar disc may be preceded by intermittent and irregular attacks of low back pain over a period of

Box 8.2

Typical findings in lumbosacral root compression producing radicular pain or a radiculopathy

L3 root compression (L2–L3 disc)

- Pain – low back, anterior or anteromedial thigh, anterior knee, sometimes groin
- Numbness – anterior thigh, knee (sometimes absent)
- Weakness – quadriceps
- Hyporeflexia – knee jerk (may be normal)
- Miscellaneous – positive reversal-leg-raising test

L4 root compression (usually L3–L4 disc)

- Pain – low back, anterior thigh, sometimes medial aspect of lower leg, sometimes groin
- Numbness – medial aspect of lower leg (may be absent)
- Weakness – quadriceps, sometimes tibialis anterior
- Hyporeflexia – knee jerk
- Miscellaneous – positive straight leg raising and reversed leg raising

L5 root compression (usually L4–L5 disc)

- Pain – low back, buttock, posterolateral thigh, lateral aspect of lower leg, lateral malleolus, sometimes dorsum of foot, sometimes groin
- Numbness – dorsum of foot, big toe, occasionally second toe or lateral aspect of lower leg
- Weakness – tibialis anterior, extensor hallucis longus, extensor digitorum brevis, sometimes gluteals
- Hyporeflexia – occasionally biceps femoris reflex
- Miscellaneous – positive straight-leg-raising test

S1 root compression (usually L5–S1 disc)

- Pain – low back, buttock, posterior thigh, calf, heel, rarely groin
- Numbness – lateral border of foot, sole, heel, sometimes fourth and fifth toes
- Weakness – gastrocnemius/soleus, gluteals, occasionally hamstrings
- Hyporeflexia – ankle jerk
- Miscellaneous – positive straight-leg-raising test

Fig 8.7 Lower lumbar and upper scaral dermatomes.

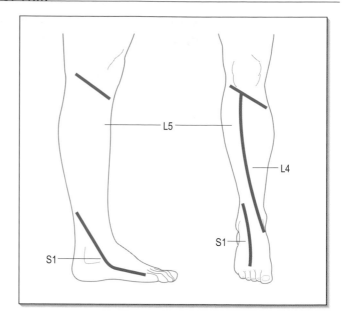

years at times, with radicular pain. Such events may have resulted in time off work, but have usually been self-limiting. The peak incidence of such episodes is between 30 and 55 years.

It is important to remember that central disc protrusion may give rise to the cauda equina syndrome, with bilateral lower limb pain, retention of urine, faecal incontinence and anaesthesia in the perianal and genital regions. This condition is a surgical emergency and urgent MRI scanning and decompression within 12 hours is essential to preserve function.

Most patients with a disc prolapse, excluding those of the cauda equina syndrome, are relieved by a short period of bed rest and symptomatic treatment with analgesics and non-steroidal anti-inflammatory drugs. After the period of rest, which should not exceed 2 to 3 weeks, mobilization is advised, and when sitting, patients should choose a firm chair with a straight back in order to avoid excessive spinal flexion. Lumbar supports, or surgical corsets, are not recommended, but rather the patient should be referred to physiotherapy where lost muscle power and tone in the lumbar region is restored. This protects the lumbar spine from excessive and abnormal movements and further attacks of pain.

When pain is not relieved by such simple measures, or when neurological signs persist, the advice of an orthopaedic surgeon or a neurosurgeon is advised. The surgeon will search for positive clinical signs of nerve root compression (sensory changes, reflex impairment and perhaps muscle wasting) and seek confirmation through the use of MRI of the lumbar spine.

In 80% of surgically treated cases, complete relief from pain and other symptoms results, and function is restored. However, in the remaining 20%, chronic pain and sensory changes persist to a variable extent and a further disc prolapse may occur. In some, infection may develop postoperatively. In others, as a result of increased stress placed on facet joints, persistent back pain develops; this may be accompanied by radiation of the pain into the posterior or anterior thigh.

When making an assessment of back pain it is useful to consider three possibilities: simple mechanical back pain, nerve root pain, and pain due to serious spinal pathology (e.g. malignancy, infection, or a non-infectious inflammatory disorder).

A careful clinical evaluation should include tests designed to exclude serious spinal disorders and they are known as 'red flags' because they indicate a high probability of abnormality.

In Chapter 5 psychosocial aspects of chronic painful disorders are described. Chronic low back pain is the most common pain disorder seen in pain clinics and there are several psychosocial risk factors mentioned in Chapter 5 that are predictors of chronicity. They are known as 'yellow flags' because of their predictive strength (Box 8.3).

Coccydynia

Pain in the region of the coccyx is relatively uncommon but, when it occurs, it often persists for months or even years. The cause is usually a fall on to the buttocks, a kick in the same region, or childbirth. It also occurs where there is repetitive strain, for example amongst rowers or cyclists who train and compete regularly. In approximately one-third of cases the cause is unknown. Diagnosis is based upon the history of injury by whatever means, rectal examination which permits movement of the coccyx and lateral radiographs taken in the sitting and standing positions, as a result of which partial dislocation at the sacrococcygeal joint may be seen. Treatment should be conservative and involve the use of a non-steroidal anti-inflammatory drug and attention to seating, which should be soft. If this treatment does not lead to improvement a local injection of a corticosteroid preparation may be effective. Unfortunately, and perhaps because of the repeated movement of the coccyx in daily life, a proportion of patients do not gain lasting relief. Surgical treatment is not advisable.

Box 8.3

Clinical characteristics of 'yellow flags': predictors of chronic pain and disability

1. Attitudes and beliefs about pain.
   (pain harmful, will increase with activity, uncontrollable, must be abolished before return to normal activities)

2. Behaviours.
   (take extended rest, withdraw from activities, avoid activity, record very high pain levels, excessive use of drugs and appliances, possible alcohol abuse, self-medication)

3. Emotions.
   (fear of pain, depression, anxiety and irritability, feeling of stress and loss of control, disinterest in social activity, feels useless)

4. Diagnostic and treatment problems.
   (dissatisfaction with treatment, lack of faith in doctors, increased visits to health facilities, seeks only physical solution, fear of chronic invalidity)

5. Other issues.
   (compensation issues, previous poor work record, negative experiences of work, overprotective family, or punitive attitudes in the family)

* The lists given in 1–5 are not exhaustive. For full details refer to Main, CJ, Spanswick, CC. In: 'Pain Management – An Interdisciplinary Approach', Chapter 4, pp. 80–83. Churchill Livingstone 2000.

The treatment of chronic pain by analgesics and the management of chronic non-cancer pain using physical techniques, e.g. local injections, radiofrequency lesions, spinal cord stimulation, are to be found in Chapter 16, and psychological techniques, e.g. cognitive/behavioural therapy, in Chapter 18.

Self-assessment questions

8.1 Which of the following statements are true?

    a. Cervical spondylosis is present in 75% of the population aged over 50.

    b. Pain due to degenerative changes in the cervical spine occurs in all those who have radiological evidence of its presence.

    c.   The most severe degenerative changes of the cervical spine occur at the levels C5/C6, C6/C7 and C7/C8.

    d.   Once present, pain from cervical spondylosis is permanent.

8.2 Which of the following statements are true?

    a.   Low back pain is experienced by 85% of adults by the age of 50.

    b.   In 50% the pain occurs for only 2 to 4 weeks.

    c.   Pain from facet joints may be experienced in the back, buttocks and thighs.

    d.   A central lumbar disc protrusion is a surgical emergency.

8.3 Which of the following statements are true?

    a.   Acute low back pain should be treated by 2 weeks' bed rest.

    b.   The relief of lumbar nerve root compression by surgery abolishes pain and sensory symptoms in the leg in 80% of patients, but a smaller number are relieved of low back pain.

    c.   Psychological factors are not important when considering prognosis in patients with chronic low back pain.

    d.   Multimodal treatment is indicated in the management of chronic low back pain where indication for surgery is absent.

8.4 Which of the following statements are true?

    a.   Red flags refer to physical signs that indicate a high probability of a significant physical lesion as the basis for back pain.

    b.   Yellow flags refer to psychological factors that predict chronic pain and disability.

    c.   Analgesic abuse is a potential risk amongst those who suffer from chronic back pain.

    d.   Radiculopathy refers to pain only in the distribution of a spinal nerve.

Local pain syndromes of the limbs

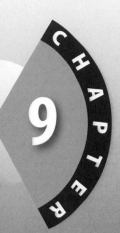

CHAPTER

9

Chapter objectives for Chapters 7 to 11

After studying these chapters you should be able to:

1 Describe the characteristic pains and associated symptoms in more common disorders of the head, face and neck, spine and limbs, thorax, abdomen and pelvis and the clinical presentation of certain generalized pain syndromes.

2 Describe the relationship between pain and a range of mental disorders.

3 Comment briefly on the overall management of pain and other symptoms in the disorders described (more detailed aspects of available management are given in Chs 14–18).

Painful shoulder

Of pains originating in the musculoskeletal system, shoulder pain is second only to back pain in its frequency. Shoulder pain results in between 2 and 4% of all consultations in general practice, whether new or repeat visits. Pain may originate in one of several sites and involve several inflammatory or degenerative mechanisms, or both, namely tendonitis, bursitis and arthritis; osteoarthritis is the most common cause of pain in the shoulder. Rheumatoid arthritis is quite common, but local infections and tumours are rare. Pain commonly arises from soft tissues around the five functional joints that comprise the shoulder. The prevalence of shoulder pain rises with age reaching almost 16% in those aged 85 years or older, in whom it is most likely to be due to degeneration in the rotator cuff.

Apart from pain arising directly from the structures forming the shoulder joint, it may also occur because of spinal pathology affecting especially the fifth cervical to first thoracic nerve roots or be referred from distal structures. Therefore, in addition to examining the shoulder and movements of the shoulder joint, there should be an examination of the neck and more distal parts of the arm, including the hand, to establish the true source of pain. Shoulder pain may occur with diaphragmatic irritation and angina pectoris.

Shoulder impingement

As a consequence of excessive use of the shoulder a bursitis, or tendonitis, may develop. The former tends to occur more commonly with increasing age and as a result of activities such as home decorating or window cleaning, involving reaching upwards and compressing muscles and ligaments around the joint forming the rotator cuff. Tendonitis occurs more often in younger people, for example those who take up sporting activities suddenly that involve the use of the shoulder. With bursitis there is a mild to severe aching pain and limitation of movement of the shoulder; with tendonitis there is pain and an associated inability to hold the arm in certain positions. The use of rest, non-steroidal anti-inflammatory drugs and perhaps a sling to support the shoulder is used to treat bursitis. Once the acute phase is over, shoulder-strengthening exercises should be undertaken. Mild tendonitis is treated by avoiding the activity that caused it, followed by paced rehabilitation. In some cases there may be a need to prescribe non-steroidal anti-inflammatory drugs and, in severe cases of both bursitis and tendonitis, injections of local anaesthetic and steroid drugs are required.

Bursitis may occur in combination with inflammation and tenderness of the tissues surrounding the joint, and this constitutes a rotator cuff tendonitis. Stiffening of the joint, especially with reduced activity, leads to a condition known as 'frozen shoulder'. Pain is provoked by certain activities, including putting on a jacket or pullover and combing or washing the hair. There is relatively little pain on palpation of the joint but pain is aggravated by internal and external rotation of the arm. The treatment is similar to that described for a bursitis or tendonitis and, as in those conditions, there should be gentle and increasing exercise.

Shoulder arthritis

There are two main sites for arthritis in the shoulder area. The first is the acromioclavicular joint and the second the glenohumeral joint where the head of the humerus articulates with the scapula. Three forms of arthritis, namely osteoarthritis, rheumatoid arthritis and post-traumatic arthritis, may affect the joints. Osteoarthritis is a degenerative disorder that is more common in the acromioclavicular and in the glenohumeral joint. The main symptom is an aching pain increased by activity and effort that worsens gradually over time. The pain from acromioclavicular arthritis is experienced at the front of the shoulder and in glenohumeral arthritis, it occurs posteriorly. Movements of the shoulder become limited by pain and wasting of the muscles occurs. In more advanced cases, pain may interfere with sleep. Crepitations may be felt by the patient and on palpation of the affected joint by the physician. Radiological examination of an arthritic joint reveals narrowing of the joint space and the formation of osteophytes in osteoarthritis, and in rheumatoid arthritis destruction of the joint occurs in the later stages of the disease.

Treatment of osteoarthritis involves reducing activity initially and controlling pain with drugs. In cases of rheumatoid arthritis drugs specific for that condition (e.g. methotrexate), or a series of corticosteroid injections, may be required. In some cases of osteoarthritis, surgical replacement of the head of the humerus in glenohumeral arthritis may be needed. In a case of an osteoarthritic acromioclavicular joint a resection arthroplasty is performed. This involves removal of the distal end of the clavicle, which allows the joint space to fill with fibrous tissue.

Rotator cuff tear

The rotator cuff consists of the muscles and tendons that surround the glenohumeral joint. A tear in the cuff may result suddenly because of an accident, or develop gradually because of occupational activities.

The presence of a tear should be suspected if the patient complains of constant pain, particularly when the arm is used for overhead activities. Pain occurs at night and prevents the patient from sleeping on the affected side. Because there is a tendency to use the shoulder less, muscle weakness develops in the muscles that surround the joint, and both the patient and the physician will detect crepitus.

Radiological examination may not reveal any obvious abnormality, but the tear may be identified using MRI, or an arthrogram.

If the tear is the result of overuse then resting the shoulder may be helpful, symptomatic relief being gained from non-steroidal anti-inflammatory drugs. Injections of corticosteroids have the disadvantage of possibly weakening the tendons that form the cuff. Once symptom control has been gained, gentle exercise should be undertaken under the supervision of a physiotherapist. In more severe cases, surgical treatment of the tear is required.

Lateral and medial epicondylitis (tennis and golfer's elbow)

In lateral epicondylitis, or tennis elbow, pain may be acute, but usually it is a chronic ache. Pain occurs at the point on the lateral epicondyle where the extensor muscles of the wrist are attached and it radiates down the lateral side of the forearm or into the upper arm, or both. The cause is a partial tear or strain of the muscle origin. Pain develops classically during grasping movements and supination of the forearm, for example when using a screwdriver or wringing wet clothes. Resistance to dorsiflexion of the wrist also increases the pain. The condition is most common in those aged between 40 and 60 years. It is self-limiting if the arm is rested, but will persist for several months if aggravated by repeated but often unavoidable movements.

Treatment of the chronic condition is by an injection of corticosteroid at the site of origin of the forearm muscles. Prior to that the use of a topically applied non-steroidal anti-inflammatory drug may give relief.

The condition of medial epicondylitis, or golfer's elbow, is characterized by pain experienced over the medial aspect of the lower end of the humerus. It is much less common than lateral epicondylitis, but the nature of the pain, its course and treatment are comparable.

Osteoarthritis (see also Ch. 11)

Osteoarthritis is a disorder of synovial joints characterized by local areas of destruction of the articular cartilage and remodelling of the subchondral bone with the formation of new bone (osteophytes) at the edges of the joint. In addition to thinning of the cartilage, cyst formation occurs in the bone underlying it. There is a mild inflammatory synovitis with thickening of the joint capsule.

Osteoarthritis of the hip and knee

By the age of 55 more than 80% of individuals have some signs of osteoarthritis on radiological examination of their joints, but only 20% experience symptoms. Given the relative insensitivity of radiology to the pathological changes that occur in joints, the use of MRI is increasingly preferred because it shows changes in subchondral bone and soft tissues.

More women are affected by this type of joint disease than men, especially with respect to osteoarthritis of the knee, whereas in men osteoarthritis of the hip is more common. The risk of osteoarthritis, especially in the knee, is increased by excess weight and the mechanical stresses placed on the joint. In established painful arthritis the pain and disability are greatest in those who are overweight. The main indications for a diagnosis of osteoarthritis are stiffness and pain in the joints, which often begins very gradually. It is especially noticeable during the first half to one hour after rising, or after sitting for some time. Joint pain is greatest after exercise and towards the end of the day. Creaking and grinding sounds, or experiences, may be reported by the patient, who is unable to put the joint through a full range of movements. In more advanced osteoarthritis painful swelling of the joint occurs, mostly because of the formation of osteophytes and, at times, because of excess fluid within the joint. Weakness of muscles around the joint develops and, as a result, it may become unstable.

Osteoarthritis of the hip may affect one or both hips causing pain, stiffness and increasing difficulty in walking. The pain is greatest during weight bearing or after exercise and is experienced mainly in the inguinal region, or on the lateral and anterior aspects of the thigh, the buttock or within the knee.

Examination reveals pain and limitation of movement, especially towards the end of movement. Crepitus will be felt in many cases on palpation of the joint.

The initial treatment of osteoarthritis of the hip is with analgesics (e.g. paracetamol or a non-steroidal anti-inflammatory drug). However, care must be taken when using the latter given the risk of intestinal ulceration, or bleeding (this occurs in 2–4% of patients who have taken a non-steroidal anti-inflammatory drug daily for a year). The patient should be encouraged to maximize their level of activity within limits imposed by the disease and, at the same time, prevent further damage to the joint, for example by weight reduction, the use of a stick, or both. Local heat and hydrotherapy may be of help. However, eventually many patients will proceed to hip replacement as their symptoms and disability increase. The outcome of this form of treatment is good in over 80% of patients who are left with a pain-free and mobile joint.

It should be remembered that chronic pain and disability, together with the limitations imposed on general activities, may well cause the onset of depressive symptoms, which require appropriate treatment.

The knee is the largest weight-bearing joint in the body and, therefore, the most often affected by osteoarthritis. When the condition develops the knee becomes stiff, painful and swollen, and this leads to considerable difficulty in walking, climbing steps and stairs, and getting in and out of chairs, or into and out of a bath. The onset of the condition is usually in the later fifties and there may be a previous history of injury to the joint – in men notably amongst those who were heavily involved in sports such as soccer and rugby. Occasionally there is a preceding history of joint surgery. The pain associated with osteoarthritis of the knee is usually experienced anteriorly and laterally. There will be a loss of muscle bulk and weakness of the muscles surrounding the joint, resulting in its instability.

Clinical examination reveals pain on movement, and especially as flexion increases. The joint may be swollen and crepitus may be detected. Confirmation of the condition is obtained by radiography or the use of non-invasive scanning techniques, or both.

Treatment of the condition in the first instance is by the use of simple analgesics as in the case of osteoarthritis of the hip. In addition, weight reduction and the use of a stick, in order to relieve weight on the joint, will be of help. However, with progress of the condition a total knee arthroplasty may be required. This is a well-established treatment and the level of pain, functional improvement, and duration of benefit is equal to that of the longer established technique of hip replacement.

Rheumatoid arthritis

(See Ch. 11.)

The main clinicopathological differences between osteoarthritis and rheumatoid arthritis are given in Box 9.1.

Pain due to vascular diseases of the limbs

Raynaud's disease

Raynaud's disease is characterized by episodes of aching and burning pain that occur chiefly in the hands and much less often in the feet or exposed areas of the face. It is associated

---

Box 9.1

Differences between osteoarthritis and rheumatoid arthritis

Osteoarthritis	Rheumatoid arthritis
• Onset in mid–later life	• Onset second and third decades (adult form)
• Symptoms confined to a few joints though process often more widespread	• Symmetrical polyarthropathy with widespread symptoms
• Inflammation rare. Erosion of cartilage, formation of osteophytes	• Inflamed synovium with destruction of all joint tissues
• Joints stiff and painful with crepitus; pain worse after activity and rest	• Joints inflamed, swollen, reddened and painful in acute phase
• Joint movements restricted	• Movements very restricted
• No systemic changes	• Non-articular changes include anaemia, fatigue, weight loss and other systemic problems
• Disability may become severe	• Disability varies in severity
• Mood changes possible	• Emotional consequences for younger person often severe

with vasoconstriction of the arteries of the extremities in response to cold or emotional stimuli. It occurs in women five times more often than in men and begins usually between the ages of puberty and 40 years.

In an attack, and in a first phase, the fingers become 'dead white', then blue as the capillaries dilate and fill with slowly circulating deoxygenated blood. Lastly the arterioles relax and the episode ends with flushing of the areas involved. During the first phase the fingers become numb and a deep aching pain of varying severity is experienced. When the hyperaemic state occurs the skin becomes red, warm, and with a severe burning pain. The duration of attacks ranges from minutes to hours, but may last for days and result in painful ischaemic skin ulcers.

The reason for the condition is unknown and abnormalities of function of the sympathetic nervous system, long thought to be the cause, have not been demonstrated. However, any factor that increases sympathetic outflow and circulating catecholamines reduces the threshold for triggering a response to the local application of cold.

Treatments include the use of vasodilator drugs at an early stage and later surgical treatments (sympathectomy) may be needed.

Erythema pernio (chilblains)

Chilblains usually occur as intensely itchy areas of skin in which a burning sensation is experienced and where the skin is reddened and sweats excessively. The chilblains are found on the lower limbs, and in particular the feet, but also on the hands. More severe cases give rise to blisters containing clear or blood-stained fluid and when that happens they resemble second degree frost bite. In the third stage full thickness skin damage occurs with local tissue death leaving necrosis, which may reach the bone; it also resembles severe frostbite.

Acrocyanosis

This is an essentially painless condition, although occasionally it gives rise to a mild ache associated with persistent blueness and coldness of the hands and feet. It is common in women during cold weather, and is often associated with the presence of chilblains.

Pain due to ischaemia and venostasis

Ischaemic pain arising from muscles is due to hypoxia in a range of disorders including atherosclerosis, thromboangiitis obliterans, arterial thrombosis and embolism. It also occurs in severe anaemia and myxoedema, hypercholesterolaemia, long-standing and heavy smoking and other less common conditions. Pain is caused by the accumulation of the products of an anaerobic respiration and it disappears rapidly when adequate oxygenation of the tissues is restored – usually by reduction in muscle work or when blood flow is increased by the use of medication. Sympathectomy has a similar result, although it leads to dilatation of skin rather than of muscle blood flow.

Treatments include the use of vasodilator drugs at an early stage and later surgical treatments involving the insertion of aortic or large vessel grafts at sites of major disease.

Chronic venous insufficiency

Dull aching pains associated with feelings of heaviness in the legs are common amongst those with varicose veins. This condition occurs in 15% of adults but is severe in only 1%. It is more common in women than in men and there is a hereditary predisposition in many. The development of dependent oedema, which disappears at night when the patient is lying flat, may develop at a later stage, as does pigmentation and eczema. Periodically, inflammatory changes leading to thrombosis in the veins produces local pain and the condition known as thrombophlebitis. Eventually the skin over the lower part of the leg becomes indurated, or thickened, and ulcerates.

The initial treatment of chronic venous insufficiency is conservative using rest with the legs elevated to relieve oedema. If the latter is more persistent it may be controlled for many months or years by the use of elasticated support stockings, which exert sufficient pressure to aid venous return. In some cases, injection or ligation of the saphenous vein may be the preferred treatment option.

Intermittent claudication and rest pain

Pain associated with exercise, albeit often no more than walking, may lead to cramp in the legs that develops because of arterial insufficiency. Pain may even occur at rest. During exercise or activity the speed with which pain develops depends on the efficiency of the arterial circulation. The distance a person is able to walk before the onset of pain in the calf or buttocks is the 'claudication distance', and because the pain disappears with rest it is known as 'intermittent claudication'. The walking distance lessens with time and the progression of degenerative changes in the arterial system.

Examination of the affected limbs reveals reduced or absent limb arterial pulses and reduced skin temperature. Murmurs and bruits may be heard in the aorta and iliac arteries.

The causes of claudication include arteriosclerosis, which commonly affects the aorta and larger arteries of the lower limbs (in addition to cerebral and cardiac vessels), and thromboangiitis obliterans, where severe or complete obstruction of arterial blood flow by atheroma occurs leading to thrombosis. Narrowing and blockage of the vessels can be demonstrated by ultrasound arteriography. The condition affects men more than women, especially in middle and older age.

Hypothyroidism or myxoedema, diabetes mellitus, hypercholesterolaemia, and long-standing and heavy smoking are associated with arterial insufficiency. Treatments include the use of vasodilator drugs at an early stage and later surgical treatments include the insertion of aortic or large vessel grafts at sites of major disease. When arterial disease is non-reconstructable, analgesia and physical treatment such as TENS, acupuncture and spinal cord stimulation may be used.

Pain of neural origin

The cubital syndrome

This condition is a radiculopathy characterized by the gradual onset of pain, numbness and sensory changes in the distribution of the ulnar nerve with, at times, weakness and atrophy of the muscles supplied by the nerve. The cause is entrapment of the nerve in the fibro-osseous tunnel formed by a groove between the olecranon process and medial epicondyle of the humerus. A myofascial covering forms a tunnel. Tinel's sign, which consists of tapping or pressing over the tunnel to provoke tingling in the distribution of the nerve, is often present. The nerve is frequently constricted and adherent. Nerve conduction studies across the elbow reveal reduced conduction time and denervation of the intrinsic muscles of the hand supplied by the ulnar nerve. The condition can be treated surgically either by decompression or by transposition of the nerve to an adjacent site. Injection directly into the tunnel must be avoided.

The carpal tunnel syndrome

This is a common condition occurring primarily in the fourth and fifth decades and especially in women. It occurs in premenstrual water retention, myxoedema, diabetes, arthritis of

the wrist joint and following fractures in the region of the wrist.
It can occur in pregnancy and in haemophilia. It is characterized by a stinging, burning or aching pain in the hand caused
by compression of the median nerve where it lies beneath the
flexor retinaculum in the carpal tunnel at the wrist. The background pain, which is a radiculopathy, is a constant ache
aggravated by activities such as knitting. Burning and stinging
pain of brief duration may be experienced in the distribution of
the median nerve and often occurs at night when it wakens
the sufferer. Tinel's sign provoked by tapping or pressing
over the carpal tunnel, or compression of the nerve by flexion
of the wrist, gives rise to a tingling sensation in the distribution
of the nerve in the hand. Clinical examination of the hand may
not reveal any evidence of abnormality but, at times, there is
decreased sensation in the distribution of the median nerve in
the palm, thumb and first two fingers, on the dorsal surface of
the tips of the index and middle fingers and on the radial half
of the tip of the ring finger. There may be weakness or wasting
of the thenar muscles, especially the adductor pollicis brevis,
with a poor grip. Nerve conduction studies are diagnostic if
they reveal delayed conduction in sensory and motor nerves
across the carpal tunnel. The condition tends to progress slowly
over a period of years and treatment is by surgical decompression of the contents of the carpal tunnel.

Postamputation pain

Postamputation pain takes two forms: phantom pain and, in
the case of limbs, pain in the amputation stump. The experience of a phantom occurs in up to 85% of limb amputees.
Phantom breast sensations and pain commonly occur after the
removal of a breast and are distressing. Phantom rectal pain
has been described. Phantom pain represents a persistence of
the body image represented in the sensory cortex. The image
persists for many months, but in many people it shrinks gradually and finally disappears. Just over 10% of cases have symptoms that are short lived. In about 3% of individuals who
undergo limb amputation a persistent and disagreeable sensation or pain is often very severe and described as a tightness or
bursting feeling, associated with the phantom. In addition,
spasms or jerking of the stump occur. Those who suffer from a
persistent and painful phantom may have certain characteristics in common in terms of the events preceding the amputation, but prediction of phantom pain is difficult. The nature of
the amputation and the patient's emotional constitution may
be relevant. Often there is a history of prolonged painful

Box 9.2

Complex regional pain syndrome I (CRPS I)

Criteria b, c and d must be present to make the diagnosis.

a. Absence of obvious damage to a peripheral nerve.

b. An initiating physical traumatic event often of a minor nature, or evidence of immobilization of the limb.

c. Constant pain, allodynia or hyperalgesia that is out of proportion to the expected consequences of the inciting event.

d. Evidence that at some time there has been oedema, an alteration in skin blood flow, or an abnormal sweating in the region of the pain.

e. The diagnosis of CRPS I is excluded if other conditions are present that could account for the degree of pain and dysfunction.

Box 9.3

Complex regional pain syndrome II (CRPS II)

All of the following criteria must be present.

a. The condition follows damage to a peripheral nerve.

b. Constant pain, allodynia or hyperalgesia that is not necessarily limited to the distribution of the damaged nerve.

c. Evidence at some time of oedema, alteration in skin blood flow, or abnormal sweating activity in the area where pain is experienced.

d. The diagnosis of CRPS II is excluded if other conditions are present that could account for the degree of pain and dysfunction.

In the light of difficulties that exist in identifying the pathophysiology underlying complex regional pain syndromes, a wide range of treatments have been tried.

The most important strategy is active physiotherapy and the encouragement of movement from the earliest time possible.

The use of antidepressants, for example amitriptyline, given its combination of analgesic and sedative properties, and anticonvulsant drugs, for example gabapentin, may help. Nerve blocks are controversial, but may help if used early. Acupuncture and TENS have been used. The evidence suggests that spinal cord stimulation may have a place in treatment as part of a rehabilitation strategy.

Pain in diabetes mellitus

The most common signs of neuropathy in diabetes mellitus are loss of tendon reflexes and vibration sense in the lower limbs. It may also give rise to a very severe burning pain in the legs and feet. At times, though, there are only pain and weakness with tenderness on gentle squeezing of the muscles. The origin of the disorder is thought to lie in the reduction of blood flow in the vascular supply of the nerves, the vasa nervorum, secondary to changes in major blood vessels. When the blood supply is barely sufficient to maintain normal function of the nerves, and local infection is present, demands of tissues for oxygen increase beyond the capacity of the local vascular system; gangrene may develop (Fig. 9.2) and the symptoms of neuropathy appear or worsen. They may sometimes be reversed by appropriate treatment of the infection. The outlook for patients with diabetic neuropathy is good if the primary condition responds well to antidiabetic therapy. In some cases, if the pain is chronic and unremitting, a depressive disorder may develop. Diabetic neuropathy may also affect other nerves, for example ocular nerves, and the nerve supply to the sexual organs and digestive tract.

Limb pain and alcoholism

Degenerative changes affecting the nervous system in chronic alcoholism are seen mostly in middle-aged men. They affect the brain, somatic peripheral nerves and the autonomic nervous system. Patients with alcoholic neuritis at an early stage of development complain of numbness, tingling, and pains in the hands and feet. The pain is often severe and burning in nature and has been described as being 'like flesh

Fig 9.2 Gangrene of the toes in a diabetic patient.

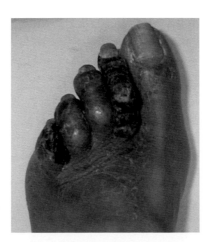

being torn from the bones'. Cramps occur in the calves, especially at night, and later both motor and sensory changes are found. Wrist and foot drop and muscle wasting may develop, especially in the periphery. Sensation is reduced and, although anaesthesia or hypoaesthesia can be demonstrated in the skin, the muscles remain painful to the touch; severe pain may be experienced if the examiner scratches the soles of the patient's feet. Tendon reflexes are diminished or lost.

The cause of alcoholic neuritis may be lack of vitamins, especially those of the B group, in the diet. Treatment involves a complete withdrawal of alcohol, rest and administration of high strength B vitamins. In mild cases, complete recovery may take place, but in those where the disorder is advanced it may take many months to disappear, or it may persist.

Neurogenic claudication

This condition, which may be mistaken for vascular intermittent claudication, is caused by stenosis of the spinal canal. Its clinical characteristic is increased pain in the legs on walking, and relief from rest, but without evidence of vascular degenerative changes. Radiological examination of the spine reveals evidence of spinal stenosis at the lumbar level.

Self-assessment questions

9.1 Which of the following statements are true?

   a. In Raynaud's disease there are marked vascular changes in the extremities with pain.

   b. Phantom limb pain is located chiefly in the residual healthy limb.

   c. In complex regional pain syndrome type I there are marked trophic changes in the skin and nails and deep pain.

   d. In complex regional pain syndrome type II there is nerve injury with deep burning pain.

   e. Intermittent claudication pain is increased by exercise and relieved by rest.

9.2 Physiotherapy is important in the treatment of which conditions?

   a. 'Frozen shoulder'

   b. Carpal tunnel syndrome

   c. Raynaud's disease

   d. CRPS type I

   e. Diabetic neuropathy

9.3 Which of the following statements are true?

    a.   Stump pain following amputation is a variant of phantom pain.

    b.   The carpal tunnel syndrome involves compression of the ulnar nerve.

    c.   'Frozen shoulder' is a term used to describe an inflammatory condition of the rotator cuff of the shoulder joint.

    d.   Shoulder pain is the second most common musculoskeletal disorder, second only to back pain.

Thoracic, abdominal and pelvic pain syndromes

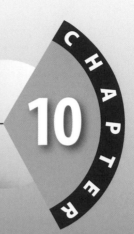

CHAPTER 10

Chapter objectives for Chapters 7 to 11

After studying these chapters you should be able to:

1 Describe the characteristic pains and associated symptoms in more common disorders of the head, face and neck, spine and limbs, thorax, abdomen and pelvis and the clinical presentation of certain generalized pain syndromes.

2 Describe the relationship between pain and a range of mental disorders.

3 Comment briefly on the overall management of pain and other symptoms in the disorders described (more detailed aspects of available management are given in Chs 14–18).

Thoracic pain syndromes

Myocardial pain

The pain of myocardial infarction is experienced as a dull, heavy, or crushing pain that is felt retrosternally and encircling the chest. It is very severe and may last several hours or until relieved by morphine. The pain sometimes radiates into the arms, particularly on the left and into the left-hand side of the neck and jaw. Alternatively, it may be experienced as no more than discomfort in the epigastric region.

The pain of a myocardial infarct is associated with marked anxiety and evidence of circulatory collapse with pallor, sweating, nausea, vomiting and marked anxiety. The blood pressure is low. The diagnosis is often by electrocardiograph (ECG) changes with the classical elevation of the ST segment and the development of Q waves. Cardiac enzymes are increased. More extensive investigations may be carried out involving the use of radionucleotide scans or coronary artery angiography, or both.

Either before or after a myocardial infarct the sufferer may experience angina caused by ischaemia of the heart muscle. It is a tight or heavy feeling within the chest that develops usually on effort, and that disappears with rest. It is the result of a workload being imposed upon the heart that is too great for its circulatory competence. For example, angina is often experienced when climbing stairs, walking up slopes or as the result of heightened emotion. Treatment is either medical or in some cases more invasive, such as radiological or surgical revascularization. Refractory angina that cannot be managed in this way may respond to stellate ganglion blockage, TENS, spinal cord stimulation, or intrathecal drug delivery. It is important that cognitive/behavioural techniques are used in parallel with this treatment to educate patients and alter their coping strategies.

Pericarditis

Pericarditis is the result of inflammation of the pericardium by a bacterial or viral infection; it may also occur after myocardial injuries. Acute pericarditis gives rise to severe pain experienced precordially, possibly with radiation to the midthoracic region, or it may resemble angina. Alternatively, pain develops in the upper part of the trapezius muscles. In some cases it is a steady crushing substernal pain, perhaps aggravated by swallowing. Leaning forward may reduce the pain. The condition results in a pericardial effusion that, if minor, causes a pericardial friction rub heard on auscultation, but with a major effusion the heart sounds are distant and muffled. In extreme cases, cardiac tamponade or compression develops and may cause cardiac arrest. Drainage of the effusion is needed.

Radiological examination of the chest reveals evidence of the effusion. An ECG examination may show ST elevation or inverted T waves. Treatment includes adequate analgesia.

Aneurysm of the thoracic aorta

An aneurysm of the aorta is a condition in which there is abnormal widening of the vessel, nowadays mainly the result of arteriosclerosis, though in the past the main cause was syphilis. The presence of hypertension is an important causative factor. The condition gives rise to deep, diffuse, central chest pain that may radiate to the midscapular region. It may be confused with angina. If the aneurysm ruptures suddenly, severe pain develops heralding a medical and surgical emergency.

Clinical examination may reveal an aortic murmur due to regurgitation, and features of acute congestive heart failure may develop. A radiological examination shows widening of the mediastinum.

Pleurisy

Sharp chest pain radiating to the arms, due to lung disease with pleural involvement, is always associated with pulmonary infarction and sometimes with pneumonia. The pain is felt deeply and in the anterior and posterior chest walls. It limits breathing.

Coughing, deep breathing and lying on the affected side aggravate pleuritic pain. There is a relationship between the site of pleuritic inflammation and the site of the pain experienced. For example, the pain is felt at the base of the chest on the affected side when inflammation of the diaphragm is present. When inflammation occurs at the apex of the chest cavity it is felt in the interscapular region. If bacteria infect the inflammatory exudate, the condition of empyema develops and pain becomes intense. Similarly, pain is severe in the presence of a pulmonary or subphrenic abscess.

In pleurisy, clinical examination reveals a pleural friction rub heard on auscultation of the chest. Definitive treatment depends on the cause, but analgesia is always needed.

Oesophageal pain

Pain due to oesophageal pathology mostly arises from its lower third because of gastro-oesophageal reflux that produces oesophagitis and possibly ulceration of the oesophagus. Reflux is often associated with hiatus hernia and, therefore, symptoms are worse when the patient is lying flat.

Pain arising from the lower oesophagus is experienced in the lower sternal region. Pain from any part of the oesophagus can be misinterpreted because it may be referred to the inter-scapular region at T6 and T7, to the neck, to the ear, to the jaw, to the precordium, shoulders, upper limbs and epigastrium. Not surprisingly it may be mistaken for a myocardial infarction. Associated symptoms may include dysphagia and regurgitation of food if an obstruction develops, as for example with a carcinoma or a benign stricture.

Diagnosis of the underlying condition depends upon the use of one or more methods of radiological and functional investigation including barium studies, motility and acid measurements, oesophagoscopy and possibly biopsy.

Pain after breast surgery

Breast surgery and reconstruction commonly cause persistent pain in the chest wall, axilla and arm on the affected side. There may be associated lymphoedema. The pain is constant and often intensified by touch and the pressure of clothing. Because of pain, the patient may not be able to tolerate a prosthesis or light clothing. Patients may experience phantom breast sensation and pain. Pain is of moderate to severe intensity and it is often not fully relieved by conventional analgesics. Simple analgesics and adjuvants such as the use of amitriptyline or gabapentin may be useful. Local preparations based upon capsaicin may be applied but require diligent and frequent use. TENS and acupuncture may help. Psychological support is often needed as the patient has to cope with both pain and the loss of the breast, altered body image and fear of persistent or recurrent cancer. Pain may occur years after a mastectomy or local removal of tumour for breast cancer with or without radiotherapy. The quality of the pain varies from moderate to severe according to the site of its origin and may indicate cancer recurrence or radiation-induced brachial plexitis. If the brachial plexus is involved the pain may be neuropathic with shooting or burning, and associated sensory changes in the limb. If deposits are found in the skeleton, in viscera, and involve the brachial plexus, survival is likely to be less than a year. Pain management depends on the aetiology of the problem.

Vertebral osteoporosis

Osteoporosis is the result of bone loss, which occurs as a normal part of ageing or, secondarily, to certain diseases or the use of particular medications (Fig. 10.1). There are other factors that increase the likelihood of osteoporosis, bone fragility and fractures. Women, especially the small boned and those of Caucasian and Asian origin, are at greater risk than men or those of both sexes from black populations. The reason for the higher incidence of osteoporosis in women is related to reduced levels of circulating female sex hormones after the menopause and, in some, there is a familial tendency to this condition. Osteoporosis is insidious in its onset and its presence may become obvious only when a vertebral fracture occurs. This may be of the compression type, as a result of which the space between vertebrae may decrease by 20–50% and result in a loss of their height. In addition, fractures of the wedge or burst variety also occur. A fracture of whatever type causes sudden severe local pain with radiation in the distribution of nerve roots, which may be compressed or distorted. Reduction in height of vertebral bodies, with or without fractures, results in an overall marked loss of height with, in some

Fig 10.1 Osteoporotic thoracic vertebra showing crush fracture and bony spurs.

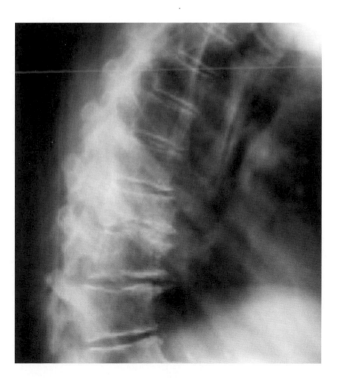

cases, the development of severe kyphosis. In this situation the patient may experience respiratory difficulties and compression of the abdominal contents.

The diagnosis of a fracture is often made by radiological means but, in addition, tests for bone density should be performed. Bone minimal density (BMD) measures are taken from the spine, hips and wrist, and low values are evidence of osteoporosis. The same technique is used to assess the rate of bone loss over time and also the efficacy of treatment.

Treatment for osteoporosis is usually non-surgical. Pain is managed by the use of simple analgesics (e.g. paracetamol), or a non-steroidal anti-inflammatory drug, but if more severe pain occurs an opioid drug of low to medium potency (e.g. codeine or dihydrocodeine) may be used. In the latter case, attention must be paid to the problem of constipation that usually accompanies the use of opioid preparations. Hormonal replacement therapy may be used, but is now not routine. Other hormonal manipulation may be used, however, due consideration must be given to the risks associated with this form of treatment and, in particular, the increased risk of stroke. There is a range of medications that slow down or prevent bone loss, including the bisphosphonates (e.g. etidronate disodium), which reduce the incidence of new fractures by 50%, and calcitonin, a non-sex hormone that slows bone loss and increases bone density, in addition to which it reduces the risk of new fractures by one-third. All patients should take calcium and vitamin D supplements. Physiotherapy may be added to the treatment plan to increase muscle strength, extend the range of motion and to increase overall physical activity, which promotes bone strengthening. In addition, it aids balance and is used to teach patients who have walking balance problems how to avoid falls. There are surgical treatments, for example vertebroplasty, but their use is for consideration only by experts.

Abdominal pain syndromes

Acute abdominal pain syndromes

Acute abdominal pain is a common medical emergency; its character is often pathognomonic of a particular condition and its treatment a matter of urgency. The most frequent causes of abdominal pain and the organs involved are given in Table 10.1 and the causes in Box 10.1, with the less common ones in Box 10.2.

Table 10.1 Common causes of abdominal pain

Viscera involved	Cause of pain
Stomach and duodenum	Hiatus hernia, gastric ulcer, duodenal ulcer
Small and large bowel	Intestinal obstruction, e.g. by tumour, bowel herniation and adhesions
	Ulcerative colitis, Crohn's colitis
	Appendicitis
	Diverticulitis
Biliary tract	Cholecystitis
	Biliary colic
Pancreas	Acute and chronic pancreatitis
Renal tract	Acute and chronic pyelonephritis
	Renal colic
	Cystitis
	Retention of urine
Female reproductive organs	Dysmenorrhoea
	Ectopic pregnancy
Infection	Chemical and bacterial
	Peritonitis

Box 10.1

Causes of acute abdominal pain in medical conditions

- Diabetes mellitus
- Acute intermittent porphyria
- Acute rheumatic fever
- Mesenteric adenitis
- Opioid withdrawal
- Abdominal migraine
- Sickle cell anaemia
- Lead poisoning
- Tabes dorsalis

Box 10.2

Uncommon causes of acute abdominal pain

Metabolic

- Diabetes mellitus
- Acute intermittent porphyria
- Lead poisoning
- Hyponatraemia
- Hypokalaemia

Haematological

- Henoch–Schonlein purpura
- Sickle cell anaemia

Neurological causes

- Multiple sclerosis
- Spinal tumours
- Tabes dorsalis (syphilis)

Pain associated with the biliary system

Biliary colic is caused by obstruction and distension of the hepatic ducts and most often by blockage of the common bile duct by biliary calculi (gallstones). Colic is experienced in the upper right side of the abdomen (the right hypochondrium), and is associated with dull pain in the back at the lower margin of the scapula. The radiation of pain occurs because the sixth to eighth thoracic nerves, which carry sensory afferent fibres from the gallbladder, also supply sensory innervation to the sixth to eighth dermatomes on the back. Small stones, or calculi, may pass into the duodenum, but larger ones result in obstruction to the flow of bile, producing obstructive jaundice.

Acute inflammation of the gallbladder, or cholecystitis, gives rise to severe and constant rather than colicky pain in the right hypochondrium. It is associated with referred pain that is experienced at the tip of the right shoulder if there is inflammation of the overlying diaphragm because its neural afferent connections via the phrenic nerve are with the third, fourth and fifth cervical segments, which also receive sensory afferent fibres from the shoulder tip area. Biliary colic and cholecystitis respond to anti-inflammatory and opioid medication.

Perforated duodenal ulcer

The pain produced by the perforation of a duodenal ulcer is experienced in the right hypochondrium and is not always preceded by an obvious history of peptic ulceration. When the peritoneum is exposed to gastric contents a local chemical peritonitis develops that becomes bacterial if not treated quickly. Perforation leads to severe pain that is focal at first, becoming more generalized. Rigidity of the abdominal muscles occurs owing to spasm because of the underlying spreading inflammatory process. Systemic effects include generalized sepsis. Occasionally, and with a small perforation, the gut contents may trickle gradually into the abdomen and down the right paracolic gutter, giving rise to pain resembling that of an acutely inflamed appendix – and possibly leading to a mistake in the diagnosis. Treatment is surgical with adequate systemic analgesia.

Acute appendicitis

Infection of the appendix, or of the mesenteric glands, is the commonest cause of pain in the right lower abdomen (right iliac fossa). Infection of the appendix is often associated with obstruction of the normal outflow of its contents, and the first signs of the disorder may be mild midabdominal colic. Inflammation of the appendix results in increased afferent activity via autonomic nerves in the tenth, eleventh and twelfth segments of the spinal cord. As a result, pain is often experienced over the distribution of those segments giving rise to central abdominal pain. Pain develops in the right iliac fossa and becomes exquisite, with increasing inflammation of the parietal peritoneum overlying the appendix. Rupture of a gangrenous appendix results in more generalized peritoneal soiling and the extension of abdominal tenderness, together with the development of rigidity involving the entire abdominal wall. Pain is experienced on rectal examination, and especially to the right. Auscultation will reveal that bowel sounds are absent. In association with the progress of inflammation, more general features of an infection develop, including low grade fever, malaise, anorexia, and flatulence, with an alteration in bowel habit in favour of constipation.

When the evidence for acute and fulminating appendicitis is equivocal, it is suggested that the patient should remain under observation for 24 hours because research has shown that this reduces the need for surgery in approximately 60% of cases.

Mesenteric adenitis

This disorder occurs primarily in children and adolescents who appear to have acute appendicitis. A clue to the presence of a mesenteric disorder is the history of a recent virus infection of the upper respiratory tract, or contact with others who have had such an infection. Those with mesenteric adenitis usually have a relatively high lymphocytosis, whereas in appendicitis there is a polymorphonuclear leucocytosis.

Records of surgical treatment for abdominal pain due to an adenitis, mistaken for appendicitis, are about 10%.

Acute pancreatitis Inflammation of the pancreas due to enzymatic autodigestion of pancreatic tissue gives rise to acute and agonizing pain that is sudden in onset and experienced in the central abdomen and mid-dorsal region. It occurs to the left of the midline in an area covered by the dermatomes of the sixth to twelfth thoracic nerves. In addition, there is rigidity of the muscles of the abdominal wall and local tenderness. In association with pain, there are signs of haemodynamic compromise with tachycardia, sometimes low blood pressure, sweating and pallor. At first the attack of pain may be mistaken for a perforated duodenal ulcer, but the serum amylase or lipase levels are usually raised in acute pancreatitis.

Acute pancreatitis occurs most often in middle-aged men and especially in heavy drinkers. An attack may be precipitated by a heavy meal or drinking bout. Acute pancreatitis occurs also when a gallstone impacted at the ampulla of Vater obstructs the main pancreatic duct. In such cases, obstructive jaundice will be present. Pancreatitis may also be seen after trauma, infections such as mumps, or be drug induced.

Acute pancreatitis is usually a self-limiting condition lasting a matter of days. Treatment is by bed rest, pain control and the treatment of systemic disturbances. Pethidine should not be used as it is too short acting, has active metabolites that may accumulate and has no advantage over other analgesics in its effect on smooth muscle. If acute pancreatitis occurs in association with alcohol consumption the patient should be advised to abstain from alcohol permanently. In some, an episode of acute pancreatitis develops into a chronic progressive disorder in which there is low grade inflammation with pain, particularly in the back, and periodic acute exacerbations. Diabetes mellitus is a complication of pancreatitis.

Acute diverticulitis Diverticulitis is a disorder of the colon that is particularly common in the elderly. With increasing age there is a tendency for small pouch-like extensions, or diverticulae, to develop in the walls of the colon and especially in its descending part. This is known as diverticulosis.

From time to time one or more of the diverticula becomes inflamed and the patient experiences dull recurrent pain, most often in the left iliac fossa. Examination reveals tenderness over the descending colon that may be palpable. The pain tends to be intermittent and to be associated with constipation. At times, during an episode of pain, the abdomen is distended. A barium enema or MRI scan will reveal evidence of multiple diverticulae.

In addition to acute abdominal pain, and possibly signs of bowel obstruction, rectal bleeding may occur. In the most severe cases, a peridiverticular abscess develops and there are more general systematic manifestations of infection, including low grade fever, malaise and anorexia.

The long-term management of diverticulosis is by the prevention of constipation, which means the use of aperients and a high fibre diet.

Chronic abdominal pain syndromes

Chronic duodenal ulcer The pain from a duodenal ulcer is experienced high in the epigastric region and the right hypochondrium, often radiating to the back at the lower margin of the left scapula. It is quite common in young and middle-aged adults. Discomfort develops 2 or more hours after a meal and is relieved by food, or the use of alkaline preparations. Symptoms of duodenal ulceration tend to be periodic, lasting for perhaps a period of days to weeks with intervals of freedom that may continue for weeks to months. It is known that often the cause of the condition is infection by *Helicobacter pylori*. If this is detected then eradication is needed.

Duodenal ulcers may give rise to medical emergencies, including bleeding and haematemesis, or more often to melaena and to perforation of the ulcer. A duodenal ulcer may be detected by barium meal examination and by the use of enteroscopy in the first part of the duodenum. When the condition is mild, and the episodes are infrequent, treatment is with antacids or, more often, by the use of an H_2-receptor blocker (e.g. ranitidine). In cases of persistent ulceration, and debilitating symptoms, given that infection with *Helicobacter pylori* is present in 45% of patients with duodenal ulcer and 70% with gastric ulcer, the prescription of two antibiotics (e.g. metronidazole and amoxicillin) and a proton pump inhibitor (e.g. omeprazole) is the treatment of choice.

Chronic gastric ulcer Patients with gastric ulceration experience diffuse pain over the upper central abdomen within a half to 2 hours after a meal. The symptoms are aggravated by eating and relieved by fasting or the use of antacids. The pain may radiate to the back. The condition occurs most often in the middle aged or elderly. Associated symptoms including nausea and, on occasions vomiting, suggests ulceration in the prepyloric region and stenosis of the outlet of the stomach. In the presence of anorexia, there may be mild weight loss. Iron deficiency anaemia may result from chronic low grade blood loss from the site of ulceration. The diagnosis of the condition is made by endoscopy, although a barium meal may be performed. It is important to take a biopsy at the time of endoscopy given the possibility that the ulcer may be malignant.

Irritable bowel syndrome

This disorder gives rise to chronic abdominal pain varying in severity over many years. It is located in almost any area of the abdomen, but is particularly common in the left iliac fossa. The pain varies from being a dull ache to a severe and, at times, colicky pain lasting minutes to hours. For reasons that are not clear, it seldom occurs during sleep. The pain is increased by eating, sometimes by drinking milk, or smoking, and perhaps by emotional stress. The pain may be relieved by defaecation, an exclusion diet or the cessation of smoking. The most commonly associated symptoms include altered bowel function in 90% of individuals who experience morning diarrhoea with five to six loose stools followed sometimes by a normal bowel movement later in the day. Alternatively the patient may be constipated and pass pellet-like faeces. Nausea without vomiting is a feature of the condition.

Examination reveals abdominal tenderness, usually over the descending colon that may be palpable, and marked tenderness on rectal examination. Pain may be experienced during sigmoidoscopy when the instrument reaches the rectosigmoidal junction. A barium enema sometimes reveals evidence of colonic spasm. Unfortunately, at times sufferers may undergo unnecessary surgery when it is believed that the condition is due to appendicitis, or a gynaecological disorder.

Standard treatment involves a diet high in roughage with the exclusion of foodstuffs only if a definite intolerance has been established. Bowel antispasmodic drugs are used. In patients with obvious psychological problems their alleviation, or resolution, is a further aspect of treatment for the disorder. If a psychological problem is suspected the clinician should seek for a history of sexual or physical abuse, depression, a high level of anxiety, or a tendency to become anxious when in stressful situations, and constant fatigue.

Crohn's disease (regional ileitis)

Crohn's disease is a chronic inflammatory granulomatous disorder of unknown aetiology that affects particularly the distal ileum, colon and less often the anus; usually in young adults. With time it may cause strictures of the small bowel and what are known as 'skip lesions' of the colon. This means that the disease develops as a series of granulomatous inflammatory patches. A proportion of patients require operative treatment with resection of an affected bowel segment that has given rise to symptoms of obstruction. Unfortunately there is a tendency for strictures to form elsewhere along the length of the bowel leading to the need for further surgery; in some cases, fistulae connecting the bowel to the abdominal wall may develop at the site of operation.

When the condition develops, the sufferer may complain initially of discomfort and distension of the abdomen, an alteration in bowel habit and weight loss. As it progresses the disease gives rise to central abdominal colic that occurs in bouts resulting from obstruction of the distal ileum. There may be abscess formation giving rise to severe and localized pain in the right iliac fossa that is constant rather than colicky in nature.

Symptoms associated with Crohn's disease where there is obstruction of the bowel include abdominal distension, nausea, vomiting and an alteration in bowel habit. In addition a mass may be palpable in the right lower abdomen and bowel sounds will be increased. The condition is aggravated by eating and is relieved by fasting. Treatment is by the use of anti-inflammatory drugs (e.g. mezalazine) as enemas or orally and, at times, corticosteroids and immunosuppression.

Pain in the genitourinary tract

Renal colic and pyelonephritis

Renal colic is a very severe colicky pain associated with nausea. It is experienced first in the loin on the affected side and radiates downwards through the right lower quadrant of the abdomen and inguinal region into the testicle, or labium. The most common cause is a renal calculus or stone, but others include clotted blood and tumour fragments. A calculus causes obstruction at the junction between the renal pelvis and the ureter, or at some point further down the ureter leading to its dilatation and to that of the renal pelvis giving rise to hydronephrosis. Eventually renal failure will occur if the obstruction is not relieved. Alternatively the calculus may reach the bladder; its passage through the ureter into the bladder causes pain and discomfort in the bladder, urgency, and frequency of micturition. The progression of symptoms occurs because the afferent nerves of kidney and ureter pass to the eleventh and twelfth thoracic and first lumbar segment of the cord that also supplies the bladder.

The immediate treatment of renal colic is intramuscular, or possibly intravenous anti-inflammatory drugs. Later treatment is by lithotripsy, which involves fragmentation of the calculus by sound waves. Alternatively, this may be done at open surgery.

Infection and inflammation of the renal pelvis gives rise to pyelonephritis, which is characterized by a severe but steady aching pain in the loin together with dysuria and signs of systemic infection including malaise, anorexia, headache, fever and perhaps rigors. Spread of the infection beyond the renal capsule gives rise to a perinephric abscess. As a result, pain extends into the inguinal and genital areas, and into the hip and thigh because the ileoinguinal and ileohypogastric nerves, together with the genitofemoral nerve, are involved in the infectious process.

The treatment of pyelonephritis is by appropriate antibiotic therapy. A perinephric abscess requires surgical intervention.

In cases of loin pain, investigations should include haematological and biochemical tests and examination of the urine for evidence of infection. Intravenous pyelogram, renal ultrasound and MRI may also be needed.

Other causes of loin pain include herpes zoster infection involving the twelfth thoracic, first and second spinal nerves. In this disorder, the appearance of vesicles associated with the infection will confirm the diagnosis. There are also musculoskeletal causes of loin pain, for example facet joint pain.

Bladder pain

Pain from the bladder is experienced suprapubically and may be the result of a distended and inflamed bladder, a bladder stone or calculus (uncommon nowadays), infiltrating tumour, or following certain forms of radiotherapy. Severe pain is experienced when the bladder contracts suddenly and involuntarily. In addition to suprapubic pain, the presence of infection or a calculus touching the trigone area leads to pain at the meatus of the urethra. The patient may experience burning pain with micturition. Small calculi may be passed through the urethra and cause a sharp burning pain in the urethra and possibly the passage of blood in the urine.

Bladder infection or cystitis is a common disorder in women. The pain is described as a diffuse low abdominal ache that changes to a burning sensation with micturition. It may be associated with low back pain and is relieved by the administration of appropriate antibiotics. Patients should also drink freely (2 litres per day). Cystitis is not common in men, but in either sex any discharge of blood in the urine should be investigated as quickly as possible. It could indicate the presence of an infection, a benign (papilloma) or malignant tumour of the bladder wall.

Prostatic pain

Prostatitis is one of the commonest urological disorders in men. It may be due to acute or chronic bacterial infection, or non-bacterial inflammatory changes. The way that the prostate gland becomes infected is uncertain, but it may be the result of ascending urethral infection or reflux of infected urine from the bladder.

The common signs and symptoms of acute bacterial infection of the prostate include raised temperature, perhaps with rigors, and pain in the rectal region, low back and/or perineal areas.

Chronic infection of the prostate is characterized by recurrent urinary infections with dysuria, and pain on ejaculation. Genital pain and haemospermia may occur. Some cases, however, are asymptomatic.

A rectal examination of the prostate when acutely infected reveals swelling, heat and tenderness, but such changes are not necessarily present in cases with chronic infection.

Acute bacterial infection requires 4 weeks' treatment with an appropriate antibiotic. In contrast, chronic infections should be treated for between 6 and 12 weeks. Recurrent infections should be treated for up to 3 months.

The prostate is the site of one of the commonest malignant tumours in men. Although the prostate itself may not give rise to pain in this condition, features of prostatism may be present and nocturia, frequency, urgency of micturition and poor control over the initiation and termination of micturition are present. Pain from secondary tumour spread, particularly to the spinal column and pelvis, may become a prominent feature of the condition.

Ectopic pregnancy

An ectopic pregnancy is a pregnancy occurring outside the uterus and the most common site is a fallopian tube. It occurs in approximately 0.25–1% of all pregnancies. Known causes include previous pelvic inflammatory disease, for example *Chlamydia* infection in young women, surgery of the fallopian tubes, a previous ectopic pregnancy (between 10 and 20% of women who have had one ectopic pregnancy will have a second), a previous termination of pregnancy, particularly if there was an infection afterwards, and in vitro fertilization.

An ectopic pregnancy is associated with a missed period, the sudden onset of acute lower abdominal pain, which is usually one sided, some irregular vaginal bleeding and a positive pregnancy test. It is important to keep the patient under careful observation because in the event of tubal rupture, signs of intraperitoneal bleeding and haemodynamic shock develop. In a proportion of patients, the pregnancy does not progress to tubal rupture, but regresses spontaneously and is slowly absorbed. The surgical treatment of an ectopic pregnancy is a matter for specialist attention.

Endometriosis

This is a disorder affecting 1–5% of premenstrual women, amongst whom it tends to appear for the first time between the ages of 25 and 35 years. Endometrial cells become implanted in tissues outside the uterus, the commonest sites being the ovaries, the fallopian tubes, the lining of the pelvic cavity, the outer surface of the uterus, and the nearby bowel. In most women, endometriosis does not cause a significant problem, and paradoxically there does not seem to be any relationship between the severity of the symptoms and the extent of the disease.

The most common symptoms are menstrual pain in the lower abdomen that begins a day or two before the start of a period, and that continues through to the end. In addition, some women report pain in the lower back, pain on micturition and on bowel movement. Patients with endometriosis complain of abnormal bleeding with heavy menstrual periods, irregular bleeding and spotting. Pain is experienced during intercourse as a result of pressure on the vagina and the cervix. There is a strong association between endometriosis and infertility.

A diagnosis of the condition is based on the history and a pelvic examination to determine whether or not implanted endometrial cells can be detected. A definitive diagnosis can be made by laparoscopy and the use of computerized tomography (CT) and MRI scanning.

Treatment depends upon the patient's age, the extent to which her symptoms cause distress and the extent of the disease. It cannot be fully eradicated without surgery, but conservative treatment may be acceptable.

Drugs used for pain include simple analgesics of the type used for menstrual pain control and non-steroidal anti-inflammatory drugs.

Various hormonal therapies are used to control endometriosis.

Dysmenorrhoea

Dysmenorrhoea is pain in the lower abdomen thought to be due to contractions of the uterus that occur when the blood supply to the endometrium is reduced. It occurs only at the completion of an ovulatory cycle. There are two forms of dysmenorrhoea: primary dysmenorrhoea, when an obvious abnormality cannot be identified, and secondary, when an underlying gynaecological disorder exists. Primary dysmenorrhoea affects more than 50% of women. In about 5–15%, the pain is severe enough to interfere with their everyday activities and it may result in absence from school or work. With age, and after childbirth, primary dysmenorrhoea diminishes.

Endometriosis is the most common cause of secondary dysmenorrhoea. The pain may be treated effectively with non-steroidal anti-inflammatory drugs or COXIBs, which should be started 2 days before the onset of menstruation and continued until the cramping pains subside. When dysmenorrhoea is more severe and interferes with normal activity, relief may be gained by suppressing ovulation.

Self-assessment questions

10.1 Match the following pain locations:
1. Shoulder tip pain
2. Severe central abdominal and mid-dorsal pain
3. Dull retrosternal pain
4. Sharp interscapular pain on inspiration
5. Pain in right hypochondrium becoming generalized abdominal pain with the diagnoses below:
   a. Myocardial infarction
   b. Pleurisy
   c. Acute cholecystitis
   d. Perforated duodenal ulcer
   e. Acute pancreatitis

10.2 Which of the following statements are true?

    a. Ectopic pregnancy occurs in approximately 10% of all pregnancies.

    b. 10–20% of women who have one ectopic pregnancy are at risk of a second one.

    c. Symptoms of ectopic pregnancy include sudden onset lower abdominal pain to left or right, a missed period and irregular vaginal bleeding.

    d. Ectopic pregnancy is not a surgical emergency.

10.3 Which of the following conditions is indicated by: recurrent heavy periods, lower abdominal pain before, throughout and after menstruation, irregular vaginal bleeding, pain on micturition, movement of the bowel during intercourse, and infertility.

    a. Dysmenorrhoea
    b. Ectopic pregnancy
    c. Endometriosis
    d. Cystitis

10.4 What diagnosis do the following symptoms suggest in a 50-year-old man: low back pain, perineal pain, dysuria, haemospermia and fever?

    a. Cystitis
    b. Pyelonephritis
    c. Prostatitis
    d. Orchitis

Generalized pain syndromes

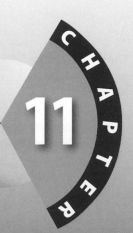

CHAPTER 11

Chapter objectives for Chapters 7 to 11

After studying these chapters you should be able to:

1 Describe the characteristic pains and associated symptoms in more common disorders of the head, face and neck, spine and limbs, thorax, abdomen and pelvis and the clinical presentation of certain generalized pain syndromes.

2 Describe the relationship between pain and a range of mental disorders.

3 Comment briefly on the overall management of pain and other symptoms in the disorders described (more detailed aspects of available management are given in Chs 14–18).

Characteristics of generalized pain syndromes

Generalized pain syndromes can arise from the joints, skeletal muscles and the components of the peripheral nervous system.

Although a number of disorders present in an acute form, most are chronic. These include some of the most difficult pain conditions to manage, given their strong association with complex, emotional and behavioural changes (Box 11.1).

Osteoarthritis (see also Ch. 10)

Rheumatological conditions afflict a large proportion of the population and are responsible for up to 10% of the total number of days lost from work because of illness each year. Osteoarthritis accounts for almost 30% and rheumatoid arthritis for about 10% of these. The causes of almost half the complaints of joint pain are unknown.

Osteoarthritis is a condition that affects central and peripheral diarthrodial joints. It is common in those that bear most weight, namely the hips, knees and feet. It occurs in the hands and occasionally in the acromioclavicular and sternoclavicular joints. It may be very troublesome if present in the temporomandibular joints. Osteoarthritis is a feature of older age and, although about 80% of the population over 55 years shows some evidence of degenerative changes in their joints, only about 20% experience symptoms. When osteoarthritis presents in early or middle life it is often secondary to damage to a joint by injury or disease. The chief symptoms of osteoarthritis are pain in, and stiffness of, the joints with loss of function that is

---

Box 11.1

Characteristics of generalized pain syndromes

- Generalized pain syndromes affect the joints of the body, the components of the peripheral nervous system and skeletal muscles singly or in combination.

- A number of the various disorders present in an acute form. Most are chronic and include some of the most difficult pain conditions to manage given their strong association with complex, emotional and behavioural changes.

- The aetiology of the conditions described in this chapter is not well understood and, as a result, treatments are aimed primarily at symptom control.

greatest after periods of immobility. There may be difficulties when walking, on rising in the morning, or after prolonged rest. The pain is aching in nature. It arises from both the joint and muscles that surround it because they develop reflex spasm. In the case of osteoarthritis of the hip, pain may be experienced in both the hip and knee because the nerves of each joint have common roots of origin. Pain is reduced when the joints are kept moving and warm. As most people are only mildly affected, symptomatic relief can be obtained from simple analgesics and non-steroidal anti-inflammatory drugs or COXIBs. These drugs should be used according to published recommendations that take into account their benefits and risks in different conditions and age groups.

Advanced osteoarthritis that causes persistent pain, sleep disturbance, poor mobility and extensive destruction of the hip or knee can be treated by joint replacement that gives excellent results in most cases. In addition to relieving symptoms arising from physical causes, this has very beneficial effects upon the patient's mental state because of pain relief and restoration of mobility. Any associated depression, anxiety, irritability and frustration tends to clear rapidly.

Rheumatoid arthritis (see also Ch. 10)

Rheumatoid arthritis is a systemic rheumatic disease that differs strikingly from osteoarthritis because there is symmetrical chronic inflammation of small joints and manifestations of a systemic nature including anaemia, neuropathies, vasculitis, with subcutaneous nodules, pulmonary and ocular problems. About three-quarters of those afflicted are between 20 and 55 years of age, with women predominating in a ratio of three to one. The onset of rheumatoid arthritis may be preceded by a physical illness, or follow a period of emotional stress. The main symptoms are pain and stiffness, warmth, redness and loss of function and strength in the afflicted joints. These include those of the hands and feet, wrists, cervical spine and temporomandibular joint. At times larger joints, for example the knees, are affected. In time, the affected joints tend to become misshapen (Fig. 11.1). The synovial tissues surrounding cartilage become thickened; these may erode surrounding tissues and bone. Aching pain predominates and it is associated with stiffness that is worse after periods of immobility, typically on wakening. It is often reduced by exercise and warmth.

Fig 11.1 Rheumatoid arthritis affecting the hand.

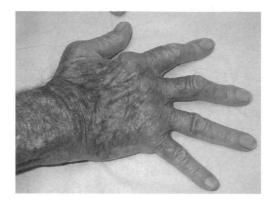

Apart from joint symptoms, and the involvement of other body systems, rheumatoid arthritis is associated with significant mental disturbances in many patients. Often they are depressed by the combined effects of chronic pain and disability, and by feelings of weakness and malaise that accompany the associated constitutional disturbances. Compared with normal people, about half of all rheumatoid patients will be depressed and, of those, 10–20% will have severe symptoms. A history of premorbid emotional problems is a predisposing factor. This chronic painful disease tends to affect young adults more than any other age group. Therefore, severe emotional problems apart from depression may occur because of the physical and social consequences of the disease. Persistent tiredness may reveal to patients that their strength and vigour have been reduced; this alters their perception of their health and self. Physical limitations restrict social activities and the patient's life pattern undergoes radical alterations that may undermine self-confidence and introduce feelings of insecurity.

Rheumatoid arthritis is a condition in which treatment by physical and psychological methods is required. The goal of clinicians is to help the patients regain their independence and mobility at home and to remain at work for as long as possible. In addition, it is necessary to maintain morale and feelings of self-worth. Sufferers need to be confident that their treatment will be both readily available and effective.

Treatment for the pain of rheumatoid arthritis involves the use of non-steroidal anti-inflammatory drugs or COXIBs. Corticosteroids, immune suppression and disease-modifying antirheumatic drugs are also used.

Acute gout

This form of arthritis is the result of a metabolic disorder. An abnormality of purine biosynthesis involving the transformation of purines into uric acid leads to abnormally high levels of uric acid in the blood and to the periarticular deposition of monosodium urate crystals. The peak incidence of the disorder is between 30 and 50 years of age and it is commonest in men.

Clinically, gout consists of a group of heterogeneous disorders. It progresses through several phases. The first is asymptomatic hyperuricaemia, the second acute gouty arthritis and the third chronic gout with the formation of tophi.

Asymptomatic hyperuricaemia is common. It is not usually treated other than by changes in diet. It is identified by the presence of an abnormally high level of serum urate without gouty arthritis or nephrolithiasis. The serum urate concentration will be greater than 416 micromoles per litre. Efforts should be made to lower the urate levels in asymptomatic patients by encouraging them to reduce the number of foods high in purines in their diet, and their alcohol intake.

Acute gout most commonly affects the first metatarsal joint of the foot, but other joints are often involved. A definitive diagnosis requires joint aspiration with the demonstration of birefringent crystals in the synovial fluid when viewed by polarized light. Treatment of this condition includes the use of non-steroidal anti-inflammatory drugs, colchicine, corticosteroids and analgesics. Non-steroidal anti-inflammatory drugs and COXIBs should be used according to recommendations. In patients amongst whom non-steroidal anti-inflammatory drugs are contraindicated, corticosteroids may be preferred. In an episode of acute gout the chief symptom is exquisite pain and the affected joint becomes swollen, red and hot. The patient may have a raised temperature and anorexia. Examination of the blood reveals an elevated erythrocyte sedimentation rate and a high serum uric acid concentration. An untreated attack will last 1 to 2 weeks. This is shortened if the patient is promptly treated in the manner described.

Tophi are chalky deposits of sodium urate that are visible radiologically; they are most common in the joints of the hands and feet and the helix of the ear. The olecranon bursar and Achilles' tendon are other classic sites for deposits, although they occur there less often. Tophaceous gout may cause a destructive arthropathy and secondary osteoarthritis. Usually it takes many years for a patient to proceed from acute gout to the condition of tophaceous gout.

Osteoporosis

(See Ch. 10.)

Fibromyalgia syndrome

The cause of this condition is unknown, but often it follows trauma or viral infection. The key feature is widespread or diffuse muscle aching pain present for 3 months or more with points of tenderness which are predictable in their location (Boxes 11.2 and 11.3). Secondly, 85% of patients complain of fatigue severe enough to disrupt their daily activities. Thirdly, over 60% experience disturbance of their sleep pattern and complain of wakening feeling tired (Table 11.1). There appears to be an association between this condition and the presence of a previous depressive illness and it should be noted that anxiety occurs in up to 72% of sufferers. The irritable bowel syndrome is reported to occur in approximately one-third of patients with fibromyalgia.

The pain of fibromyalgia is a deep ache. It is located in the muscles and most often in those of the neck, shoulders, chest and lumbar regions. Other changes occur in the more distal parts of the limbs, including aching, with swelling, stiffness and numbness. Although the pain is continuous its focus moves from day to day.

Tenderness on pressure over tender points gives rise to marked pain locally. Trigger points are found within the muscles, over tendon origins and over bony prominences. Palpation elicits pain and a reactive hyperaemia develops both at the tender site and in the areas to which pain is referred. In 60–70% of those afflicted the condition is aggravated by cold,

---

Box 11.2

Fibromyalgia syndrome

- Pain distribution widespread including both sides of the body, above and below the waist, together with pain in the cervical spine, thoracic or lumbar spine and chest.
- Pain should be present in at least 11 out of 18 sites where muscle points can be identified by palpation that is described by the patient as painful.
- Pain must have been present for a minimum of 3 months.

Box 11.3

Eighteen tender points in diagnosis of fibromyalgia syndrome

Definition. Pain on digital palpation must be present in at least 11 of the following 18 tender point sites:

- Occiput: bilateral, at the suboccipital muscle insertion
- Low cervical: bilateral, at the anterior aspect of the intertransverse spaces at C5–C7
- Trapezius: bilateral, at the midpoint of the upper border
- Supraspinatus: bilateral, at origins above the medial border of the scapular spine
- Second rib: bilateral, upper surfaces just lateral to the costochondral junctions
- Lateral epicondyle: bilateral, 2 cm distal to the epicondyles
- Gluteal: bilateral, in upper outer quadrants of buttocks in anterior fold of muscle
- Greater trochanter: bilateral, posterior to the trochanteric prominence
- Knee: bilateral, at the medial fat pad proximal to the joint line.

  Digital palpation should be performed with a force of 4 kg.

  For a tender point to be considered 'positive' the subject must state that the palpation was painful; 'tender' is not to be considered 'painful'.

  Note: For classification purposes, patients will be said to have fibromyalgia if both criteria are satisfied. Widespread pain must have been present for at least 3 months. The presence of a second clinical disorder does not exclude the diagnosis of fibromyalgia.

humid weather, fatigue, anxiety or more general mental stress. Prolonged or vigorous work increases the severity of symptoms, and warmth and rest temporarily reduces them.

Relief of the condition is mainly symptomatic given that its cause is not fully understood. It involves an explanation to the patient about its nature. Physical treatment includes the use of low doses of amitriptyline (5–50 mg) at night. Non-steroidal anti-inflammatory drugs and steroid preparations do not appear to be of any assistance. Cardiovascular fitness training, the use of cognitive/behavioural therapy or biofeedback is strongly recommended to help patients cope with their symptoms.

Table 11.1 Percentage frequency of symptoms in patients with fibromyalgia syndrome

Symptoms	%
Pain	94
Fatigue	85
Stiffness	76
Anxiety	72
Poor sleep	62
Generalized aching	60
Mental stress	60
Swelling	40
Depression	37
Paraesthesia	36

Myofascial pain syndrome

Various synonyms are applied to this condition including fibrositis, myalgia, muscular rheumatism and non-articular rheumatism. It occurs three times more often in women than in men. The criteria for the classification of the myofascial pain syndrome were proposed by the American College of Rheumatology in 1990 (Box 11.4).

The myofascial syndrome commonly accompanies autoimmune rheumatic and non-rheumatic disorders, such as rheumatoid arthritis and Sjögren's syndrome, Raynaud's phenomenon and hypothyroidism. The condition shows marked differences in presentation compared with fibromyalgia (Table 11.2). The condition tends to be chronic, and the cause is unknown. It occurs frequently after trauma, for example after a whiplash injury, or other musculoskeletal injuries.

Myofascial pain syndrome occurs in one voluntary muscle, or a small group of voluntary muscles, that are found to be tense, shortened and painful, if stretched passively or strongly contracted voluntarily. Trigger points are to be found in the muscle. Palpation reveals them to be 'taut bands' that feel like either a firm band or a nodule. This, when stimulated by pressure, twitches and is painful; pain often is referred more widely. The cause of the condition in the muscle may be nerve root irritation, and therefore this should be investigated. The treatment of this condition depends on its duration and the almost certain development over time of marked associated emotional

Box 11.4

Clinical criteria for the diagnosis of myofascial pain syndrome

Major criteria

1 Regional pain complaint.

2 Pain complaint or altered sensation in the expected distribution of referred pain from a myofascial trigger point.

3 Taut band palpable in an accessible muscle.

4 Exquisite spot tenderness at one point along the length of the taut band.

5 Some degree of restricted range of motion, when measurable.

Other criteria

1 Reproduction of clinical pain complaint, or altered sensation, by pressure on the tender spot.

2 Elicitation of a local twitch response by transverse snapping palpation at the tender spot or by needle insertion into the tender spot in the taut band.

3 Pain alleviated by elongation (stretching) the muscle or by injecting the tender spot.

Table 11.2 Some differences between fibromyalgia and myofascial pain syndromes

	Fibromyalgia syndrome	Myofascial pain syndrome
Sex	Female/male 10 : 1	Male/female 2 : 1
Tender point pain	Local	Referred
Tender point distribution	Widespread	Regional
Tender point anatomy	Muscle–tendon junction	Muscle belly
Stiffness	Widespread	Regional
Fatigue	Debilitating	Usually absent
Treatment	Drugs	Local injection Stretch and spray therapy
Prognosis	Seldom cured	Usually good

and behavioural changes. Tender trigger points may be injected with local anaesthetic, corticosteroid, hypertonic saline or botulinum toxin. Gentle massage and passive stretching of the muscle should follow this. Other forms of treatment include the use of TENS, acupuncture, acupressure or the use of a cold spray or pack on the trigger point, with associated passive stretching of the muscle. This is known as the 'spray and stretch technique'.

As in the case of the fibromyalgia syndrome, the use of cognitive/behavioural therapy and relaxation techniques may be of help.

Self-assessment questions

11.1 In which of the following are these signs and symptoms detected: acute pain, local swelling, local heat, and crystals in synovial fluid?

a. Rheumatoid arthritis

b. Gout

c. Tuberculous infection of a joint

11.2 Pain present in 11 of 18 sites in the body, pain within muscles, together with fatigue, anxiety, depression and poor sleep are features of which of the following?

a. Myofascial pain syndrome

b. Fibromyalgia

11.3 Which of the following are used in the treatment of rheumatoid arthritis?

a. Aspirin

b. Non-steroidal anti-inflammatory drugs

c. Corticosteroids

d. Colchicine

e. Gold injections

11.4 Which of the following are hazards when using COX-1 non-steroidal anti-inflammatory drugs in the elderly?

a. Drowsiness

b. Renal damage

c. Glaucoma

d. Gastrointestinal bleeding

e. Platelet abnormalities

Pain and mental disorders

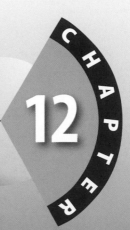

C H A P T E R

12

Chapter objectives

After studying this chapter you should be able to:

1 Understand and define the term mental disorder.

2 Identify mental disorders that include pain as a symptom.

3 Identify mental disorders, and disorders of behaviour, that may occur during painful illnesses or after injury.

Pain and the emotions

A change in emotion and behaviour is an inevitable response to pain. Acute pain tends to evoke anxiety, and persistent pain generates, in addition, depression of mood and more complex psychological changes of emotion and behaviour. Also, pain occurs as a feature of certain mental disorders in the absence of obvious tissue damage resulting from injury or disease. The resulting disorder is usually mood related, or one of the somatoform group; both are described in more detail later.

The classification of psychiatric disorders is based upon groups of psychological, and often physical, symptoms that occur in clusters with a high degree of predictability. As such, they have implications for treatment, and for prognosis. However, sometimes the boundaries between different disorders are not clear, as occurs at times with schizophrenia and manic disorder. Certain mental disorders show a familial tendency indicating that genetic factors are important determinants. In the last half-century, and particularly more recently, other biological clues about the origins of some mental disorders, particularly those in the affective and schizophrenic groups, have been inferred by observations on the effects of psychotropic drugs, like the antidepressants and antipsychotics. More recently still, evidence has started to appear as a result of non-invasive scanning techniques that allow evaluation of the metabolic functions and blood flow within areas of the brain concerned with cognitive/emotional control. Biology is not the only reason, however, because psychosocial and environmental factors often play a part in their appearance; the seed is present but needs to be nourished.

The criteria used in the diagnosis of mental disorders are described in 'The International Classification of Diseases', published by the World Health Organization, now in its tenth revised edition and in 'The Diagnostic and Statistical Manual of the American Psychiatric Association', which is in its fourth and revised version. They are known respectively as ICD-10 and DSM IV-TR. Both describe diagnostic criteria and the DSM IV-TR provides, in addition to diagnostic features, information about associated features and disorders, cultural, age- and gender-related factors regarded as important, together with alternative diagnoses and information of an epidemiological nature. Treatment guidelines are also given.

Questionnaires and checklists, for example the Leeds Depression and Anxiety Scale and the Beck Depression Inventory, have been devised to aid diagnosis. Standardized interviews increase the reliability of diagnoses.

Physical illness and pain

Chronic diseases in general, and painful conditions in particular, are associated with an increased prevalence of psychiatric diagnoses. This is known as psychiatric comorbidity. The stress of living with pain appears to be the main factor leading to the development of depression in particular, and not a premorbid personal or family history. However, those with such a history develop depression sooner than those without it and so a degree of vulnerability does seem to exist. Patients who have chronic pain with comorbid psychiatric symptoms have greater functional impairment and should be viewed as having a more uncertain outcome, both in terms of pain and disability, and of their psychiatric condition.

Studies of patients attending all forms of pain clinics, the great majority of whom have chronic pain, have revealed that up to 70% have emotional problems ranging from minor ones to the most severe. The most common emotional changes are depression, with or without anxiety, or anxiety alone. Studies of patients with chronic persistent pain versus intermittent pain reveal that, of the former, 18% have moderate to severe depression compared with 8% of the latter. Studies of those over 65 years of age reveal that patients with persistent illnesses or disabilities are at increased risk of the onset of a depressive disorder. For example, in up to 10% it will be severe, and the overall prevalence is in the region of 25%.

Mood disorders and pain

The psychiatric symptoms of a major depressive episode are given in Box 12.1. It should be remembered that those who have physical illness often experience tiredness, poor concentration, and an altered sleep pattern. In addition their appetite may be reduced resulting in a loss of weight. These symptoms are frequently part of a depressive syndrome also, therefore it is very important in the physically ill to make an accurate assessment of mood, searching for evidence of persistent feelings of depression, a reduction or loss in capacity for enjoyment, feelings of guilt, indecisiveness, despair and suicidal thoughts. The timing of the onset of depression may be an aid to diagnosis. In those who have physical illnesses, depression

Box 12.1

Symptoms of a major depressive episode

- Low mood
- Loss of interest
- Reduced self-confidence and self-esteem
- Ideas of guilt or unworthiness
- A bleak and pessimistic view of the future
- Ideas or acts of self-harm
- Diminished activity, reduced energy, and increased fatigue*
- Reduced concentration and attention*
- Disturbed sleep/early waking*
- Diminished appetite and weight loss*
- Loss of libido*
- Loss of pleasure in usual activities*

* Common to physical illness and depression.

usually develops weeks or even months after the onset of the physical symptoms, whereas pain arising as a symptom of a depressive disorder tends to develop almost at the same time as the change in mood. In some patients the pain is experienced at the site of a previous injury, or where there has been surgical trauma (appendicectomy or tooth extraction), and this may well deflect the doctor from making a correct diagnosis of a mental rather than a physical condition.

It has been suggested that there are mechanisms by which emotional changes give rise to pain of a psychological rather than a physical disorder that, at times, may be so severe as to deflect the physician from a correct diagnosis. Amongst the hypotheses proposed are the following:

1 The presence of certain personality traits and, in particular, a tendency to feel guilt, resentment and hostility easily. Individuals with these characteristics may have a history of high levels of medical consultations and multiple somatic complaints. They may have a history of frequent surgical procedures.

2 It was suggested in the 1950s, and on the basis of personality traits of the type described, that individuals who adapt to difficulties in life via traumatic, social or personal relationships, e.g. failed marriages, or the development of a masochistic role in the relationship may, in addition, have

complaints of persistent pain that do not have an obvious physical cause.

3 Experience of sexual and physical abuse in early life, and the management of personal relationships through violence, has been linked with the development of chronic pain in later life.

Recent studies of individuals with the characteristics described have not yielded evidence that there is a close relationship between these characteristics and chronic pain in adult life, with the possible exception of the early experience of physical and sexual abuse.

Anxiety and pain

Pain is a common comorbid factor with a range of conditions associated with the presence of anxiety. Anxiety is a common experience and in one study 25% of the general population in the United States admitted to having suffered from severe anxiety at some time. Pain occurs in several anxiety disorders, including general anxiety disorder and post-traumatic stress disorder.

General anxiety

Feelings of anxiety and tension are a common and normal part of everyday life. They may increase to the point where the feeling becomes sufficiently intense and prolonged to result in a psychiatric disorder known as 'general anxiety disorder' (see Box 12.2). In those in whom anxiety arises as a result of stresses of everyday life (e.g. work or family problems and financial difficulties), pain may develop and does so most often in the form of headache, facial, neck, head, chest or back pain. Pain of this type may be very severe and be associated with a fear of catastrophic illness such as, for example, a brain tumour or heart attack, or be an aspect of a stress-related illness, like the irritable bowel syndrome.

Post-traumatic stress disorder

Post-traumatic stress disorder is a specific anxiety disorder that embraces the emotions, cognitions, and behavioural consequences of trauma that, though it may not cause injury, is of terrifying proportions and carries with it the threat of death to the person, or the actual death or threat of it to others. The condition commonly develops as a result of motor accidents, train crashes, mining accidents, building collapses and other

Box 12.2

Symptoms of a generalized anxiety disorder

- Excessive anxiety and worry most days for a minimum of 6 months.
- Difficulty in controlling the worry.
- Irritability.
- Difficulty in concentration, mind goes blank.
- Muscle tension.
- Easily fatigued.
- Sleep problems, difficulty in getting to sleep, frequent wakening.
- Waking exhausted.
- Significant impairment of functions of daily life.

sudden and terrifying events. The symptoms include the reliving of the event itself at frequent intervals as recurrent and intrusive recollections and dreams. There is intense psychological distress on exposure to internal or external cues that symbolize or resemble an aspect of the trauma and, in association with them, there will be physiological reactions associated with anxiety, including palpitations, sweating and breathlessness. These experiences occur especially on wakening from distressing dreams, or after seeing or hearing some event that reminds the person of the accident. Those who have post-traumatic stress disorder tend to avoid stimuli that arouse thoughts or visions of the trauma, and their level of emotional response to others is numbed. They have persistent symptoms of arousal, including major disturbances of sleep pattern, as a result of which often they sleep only for 1 or 2 hours a night for many months. Frequently they are very irritable and anxious. In order to make the diagnosis of post-traumatic stress disorder the symptoms described above must be present for at least 1 month, be distressing and result in impaired social, and/or occupational, functions (Box 12.3). The symptoms described are surprisingly common in pain clinics and have been recorded in as many as 35% of people who have suffered injuries.

Somatoform disorders and pain

A somatoform disorder is one in which psychological problems are manifest as physical ones through the process of somatiza-

---

Box 12.3

Post-traumatic stress disorder

- Exposure to a traumatic event that results in death, a threat of death, or serious injury, or a threat to the physical integrity of the self. There are associated feelings of intense fear, helplessness, or horror.

- Recurrent intrusive thoughts, dreams, or feeling that the event is reoccurring, are experienced frequently. The experiences take the form of 'flashbacks', which are associated with intense distress and perhaps sweating and tremor, either spontaneously, when wakening from sleep, or when stimulated by an event that symbolizes the original trauma.

- Stimuli associated with the traumatic event are avoided, there is numbing of emotional responses to others and social withdrawal.

- Sleep is reduced to short periods (1–3 hours) with distressing dreams, the individual is very irritable, unable to concentrate, is easily startled and is hypervigilant.

(The symptoms described in the second to fourth bullet points must be present for a minimum of 1 month for the diagnosis to be made.)

---

tion. The majority of patients do not connect their physical symptoms with their psychological problems. Somatization is a normal rather than a pathological process unless it takes an extreme form.

Pain is a common aspect of somatization, but is generally transient and only two categories, hypochondriasis and pain disorder, have pain as a major symptom (hypochondriasis), or as the main symptom (pain disorder).

Hypochondriasis

Individuals with hypochondriasis are preoccupied with the thought, or the belief that, they have a serious disease, but without corroborating medical evidence (see Box 12.4).

Hypochondriasis is associated with high levels of anxiety and those who suffer from it seek medical opinions and reassurance repeatedly and are often referred to specialists. As a result, often they undergo unnecessary investigations. Reassurance usually brings relief, but those who are severely affected have persistent symptoms and seek further investigations. Hypochondriacal complaints may take the form of worries

Box 12.4

Hypochondriasis

- Raised somatic awareness/preoccupation with bodily functions.

- A fear of disease.

- An unshakeable belief on the part of patients that they have a serious and possibly life-threatening illness for which evidence cannot be found.

- The belief of the presence of disease may be of delusional intensity and be a symptom of a psychiatric disorder, e.g. depression, schizophrenia. (The delusion is a false belief held with convictions for which there is no evidence in reality. It is not in keeping with cultural beliefs.)

about minor breathing problems, skin irritations, sore throats, and minor aches and pains. Those who have a more severe form may experience chest pains and believe that this represents heart disease, or headaches that represent a brain tumour.

Individuals who suffer from hypochondriacal traits are more likely than others to have had serious illnesses earlier in life, or have been close to family members who have had such illnesses, at times ones that are painful. Hypochondriacal traits, present early in adult life, and tend to intensify with age as bodily functions begin to fail and family and friends die.

The treatment of mild hypochondriasis is by reassurance and minimal investigation other than general examination. Every effort should be made not to reinforce the patient's anxieties. Hypochondriacal thoughts and beliefs of a delusional nature occur as aspects of mental disorders, such as depression and schizophrenia where the treatment is of the primary condition.

Pain disorder

Individuals who have pain disorder may or may not have a history of a physical cause for pain at one or more sites and, should there be a physical cause, it is generally minor. In contrast, the level of disability due to pain is high. Psychological factors play a significant role in the onset, severity, exacerbation or maintenance of the pain (Box 12.5). Unlike patients with hypochondriasis, the individual with pain disorder does not have a fear of disease or injury, but a belief that there must be a cause for pain of a physical nature, and this conviction leads

Box 12.5

Characteristics of pain disorder

- Pain in one or more anatomical sites is the predominant focus of the clinical presentation and is of sufficient severity to warrant clinical attention.
- The pain causes clinically significant distress or impairment in social, occupational or other important areas of functioning.
- Psychological factors are judged to have an important role in the onset, severity, exacerbations or maintenance of the pain.
- The symptom or deficit is not intentionally produced or feigned (as in fictitious disorder or malingering).
- The pain is not better accounted for by a mood, anxiety or psychotic disorder, and does not meet the criteria for dyspareunia.

Acute pain disorder – less than 6 months' duration.
Chronic pain disorder – more than 6 months' duration.

them from one doctor and one clinic to another to seek a cure. The level of disability is usually considerable and out of keeping with any physical problem that may be detected. It disrupts the patient's whole life. Most will have stopped work and many take significant amounts of analgesics and may even have become dependent upon them. Their family lives have been altered so that they have become dependent on others to a great extent. If feelings of depression or anxiety are present, and at the level of a formal psychiatric disorder, the diagnosis of pain disorder cannot be made.

The most common sites for pain are the lower back, or the lumbar region, and the face. Symptoms have usually been present for many months, and often for years, when patients are referred for assessment at a pain clinic. They are likely to have undergone many clinical investigations and different forms of treatment, which sometimes includes surgery. Treatment by physiotherapy may have been tried unsuccessfully on several different occasions.

The possible origins of pain in pain disorder are becoming clearer. It is known that acute pain, though it may be quite trivial, leads to changes in mechanisms in the spinal cord that modulate pain. The changes that occur lead to persistent pain, although any peripheral tissue injury may have long since disappeared. It is more difficult to explain this change if there has not been a history of injury, but there is a growing belief that alterations in the functions of the pain modulating mechanisms of the spinal cord may develop as the result of changes in brain function and give rise to pain without evidence of peripheral pathology.

The management of the condition is by a combination of cognitive and behavioural treatments, physical therapy, and often detoxification from powerful narcotic drugs, most often dihydrocodeine. The aim of a multidisciplinary programme is rehabilitation; this does not mean the restoration of perfect health and freedom from pain, but the improvement of physical function, the abandonment of unnecessary rest, the restoration of more normal relationships and roles within the family, and the cessation of the misuse of analgesic drugs. In addition, the programme is designed to reduce medical consultations and investigations and so to avoid re-establishing the previous pattern of behaviour that led to unnecessary investigation and treatment. Such programmes require the help of those who are highly experienced in the management of pain patients because, given their intense focus upon a physical cause for pain, the person with pain disorder does not readily accept that the condition cannot be completely relieved and that the best way forward is through a programme of rehabilitation.

Personality disorder and pain

Individuals who have a disorder of personality show an enduring pattern of mental activity and behaviour that deviates markedly from the expectations of the culture in which they live (Box 12.6). For example, their ways of perceiving and interpreting themselves and other people and events, the range, intensity and appropriateness of their personal responses, together with the way in which they interact with others and the control of basic impulses, are outside the normal range. Ten specific personality disorders are known to psychiatrists; however, they are not discussed in this book individually and should more information be required the reader is referred to a psychiatric textbook. A surprisingly high proportion of patients with chronic pain had been found to have at least one form of personality disorder and those of the antisocial, borderline and paranoid type are amongst the most common. The presence of such a disorder is associated with the poor prognosis for the physical condition and a higher relapse rate than amongst people who do not have it. In addition, pain tends to intensify pre-existing pathological personality traits resulting in poor ability to cope with pain, with extension of the pain problem

Box 12.6

Personality disorders

- Personality disorder is characterized by personality traits that are pervasive, inflexible and maladaptive. They cause significant functional impairment or subjective distress, or both.

- A personality disorder is an enduring pattern of inner experience, and behaviour, that deviates from the expectations of the individual's culture.

- The onset of personality disorder occurs in adolescence or early adult life. They are stable over time.

- There are 10 types of personality disorder, each of which has specific diagnostic criteria. Some examples include: paranoid, schizoid, antisocial, histrionic and dependent disorders.

For more detailed information the reader should consult the Diagnostic and Statistical Manual of Mental Disorders – 4th edn (DSM-IV-TR) published by the American Psychiatric Association in 2000.

and less successful treatment. Despite what is said above there is no reliable association between any specific type of personality disorder and pain, or a poor response to its treatment.

To conclude, personality disorders and major psychiatric illnesses are associated with greater vulnerability to pain and disability and the presence of either or both is associated with a poorer prognosis.

Adjustment to disease and injury

Those with more than a minimal injury, or minor disease, may have to make adjustments in their lives to accommodate for pain and disability. In some, however, the level of distress is far in excess of what would be expected in the circumstances and the level of impairment is similarly exaggerated. Unlike the condition of pain disorder this situation arises as a response to a well-defined physical event and is known as an adjustment disorder (see Box 12.7). It occurs as a reaction to illness and injury and to a variety of social problems including job losses, marital strife and a reduced income.

The level of disability, or failure to cope, is thought to be linked to anger and distress suffered by people who see their goals in life destroyed, their income reduced, and their family

Box 12.7

Characteristics of adjustment disorders

1 The development of emotional behavioural symptoms in response to an identifiable stressor(s) occurring within 3 months of the onset of the stressors.

2 These symptoms or behaviours are clinically significant as evidenced by the following:

  a. Marked distress that is in excess of what would be expected from exposure to the stressor

  b. Significant impairment in social or occupational (academic) functioning.

3 The stress-related disturbance does not meet the criteria for another specific mental disorder and is not merely an exacerbation of a pre-existing mental or personality disorder.

4 The symptoms do not represent bereavement.

5 Once the stressor (or its consequences) has terminated the symptoms do not persist for more than an additional 6 months.

  An acute disorder does not exceed 6 months in duration.
  A chronic disorder exceeds 6 months.
  The predominant symptoms of an adjustment disorder may be:

  a. Depressed mood

  b. With anxiety

  c. With anxiety and depressed mood

  d. With disturbance of conduct (antisocial behaviour)

  e. With mixed disturbances of emotions and conduct.

and social life impaired, by an injury or disease that they may blame on others. It is clear that the person with an adjustment disorder cannot come to terms with the fact that, as a result of the injury or disease, they will have to give up their job and retrain for alternative employment, should that be available. There is a 'denial of disability'. The emotional content of the reaction varies and may take the form of anger, depression, anxiousness, or a mixture of all three. In some cases, disturbances of behaviour accompany the emotional disorder resulting in aggressive or antisocial behaviour often linked to excessive consumption of alcohol. The presence of an adjustment disorder is associated with increased complaints of pain, the disruption of the treatment of any underlying condition and its prolongation. However, it is usual for signs of the disorder to disappear within 6 months, once the underlying stress has been resolved, and acceptance of any disability that is likely to be permanent has been achieved. At that point, pain arising from the disease, or disorder giving rise to the condition, is more readily treated by counselling but, in some cases, cognitive/behavioural therapy is required. If depression is present the use of antidepressant medication should precede cognitive behavioural therapy.

Self-assessment questions

12.1 Which of the following statements are true?

a. More than 75% of patients attending pain clinics have emotional problems.

b. The prevalence of depression in those over 65 years of age and with persistent illness or disabilities is 25%.

c. Symptoms of post-traumatic stress disorder are present in up to 35% of patients attending pain clinics.

d. There is a direct correlation between specific forms of personality disorder and greater vulnerability to pain and disability.

12.2 When dealing with patients who suffer from painful and disabling disorders it is important when considering a possible diagnosis of a major depressive disorder to identify symptoms diagnostic of that condition. Which of the following are *specific* for major depressive disorder:

a. Diminished appetite

b. Ideas of guilt and unworthiness

c. Reduced self-confidence and self-esteem

d. Diminished activity, reduced energy, and increased fatigue

e. Low mood

f. A bleak and pessimistic view of the future

Pain management

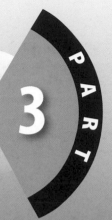

3

PART

The examination of
patients with pain

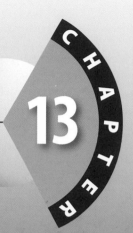

13

Chapter objectives

After studying this chapter you should be able to:

1 Understand and be able to use a comprehensive
   method for the examination of patients in pain.

2 Know how to use the outcome of your
   examination to plan treatment for your patient.

3 Be aware of when to seek the advice of a pain
   specialist team or when to refer a patient to a pain
   management clinic.

Examination of the patient and basic principles of pain management

A full medical history and examination, with particular emphasis upon pain, is essential for the assessment of painful disorders. Physical, psychological and social information must be obtained. It is advisable to seek corroboration from a close relative or friend of the patient; this is particularly important in patients with chronic pain. The examination should be supported by tests that provide specific information about the location and nature of the pain (pain drawing), and the severity of the pain (VAS, PPT and SF-MPQ – see Ch. 3). These measures are particularly useful when a period of treatment is envisaged with a need to evaluate its effects. A full drug history should be taken to establish the value of existing treatment and the possibility of multiple drug intake, including 'over-the-counter drugs', with the dangers of drug toxicity. There is a need to establish any evidence for problem drug use. After initial screening, other clinical specialists may need to conduct examinations specific to their areas of skill in order to formulate a full assessment and management plan.

Questions to ask about pain

Always begin by asking directly about the pain. This convinces patients that you believe they have pain because others may have given a different impression.

Physical questions about pain

1   What is the location of pain, its duration, and estimate of severity overall? Ask the patient to rate the pain on a scale of 0–10 (see Ch. 3).

2   Is there any known reason for the onset of pain (e.g. trauma, illness, etc.)?

3   Does the pain vary with changes in posture, other movements, or time of day? Does it affect sleep?

4   How does the pain affect function and daily activity? What can the patient do when the pain occurs? What can the person not do?

5   What is the effect of medication on pain? What pain medicines are being taken – analgesics, antidepressants, anticonvulsants, or other treatments? Is there evidence of problem drug use? Which medication is most effective? What side effects are present? Is there any possibility of adverse drug interactions?

6   What has been the effect of other forms of treatments for pain – surgery, injections of various kinds, use of stimulation techniques, physiotherapy, acupuncture, and strategies used by chiropractors, osteopaths, hypnotherapists or psychologists?

Psychological questions about pain

A second set of questions concerns emotional aspects of pain. This should not be a difficult issue if the clinician has started by accepting that pain is present and after stating that being in pain changes emotions and feelings.

1   Have emotional changes been experienced – tension, anxiety, fear, panic, depression or anger? Explore each in terms of the timing of the onset of the emotional change in relation to the onset of pain, and the severity of pain in relation to the extent of the emotional disturbance. For example, pains tend to be more severe when tension and anxiety are high and when depression is present.

2   Determine what psychological factors, if any, reduce pain and, in particular, rest and relaxation, psychotropic drugs and psychological methods of treatment.

3   Determine whether or not there are causes of emotional distress in the patient's life that may be associated with pain – problems in the family, in relationships, at work and with money (see questions 1 and 2). The presence of background stresses often reduces coping ability and may even enhance pain severity.

4   Does the pain affect relationships and sexual function?

5   Determine whether or not the patient has a history of an emotional disorder of any description, note its nature, when it occurred, and whether or not it was associated with the presence of pain. A very recent period of emotional disorder may leave the person emotionally vulnerable and less able to cope with pain.

6   What pattern of behaviour does the patient show with respect to self-management of the pain – does the person rest and, if so, how long and how often? How well does the patient set achievable goals and pace him or herself?

7   What drugs does the patient take for pain – including those from a doctor and those bought over the counter? Are drugs being taken to excess?

Social questions about pain

1   What have been the consequences of the painful disorder for the patient's home life, family relationships and usual domestic and social activities? What level of dependency has been established? To what extent has the individual withdrawn from work?

2   Have financial problems of any description developed during the course of the pain condition?

3   What effect, if any, has the pain had on the individual's personal habits; the level of alcohol consumption and the amount of tobacco smoked? Have non-prescribed or 'street drugs', or both, been used and, if so, what is the effect upon pain?

Specific pain assessment measures

Having completed a full pain interview it may be supplemented by the use of the following (for details of items 1–4 see Ch. 3):

1   The pain drawing

2   The Visual Analogue Scale (VAS) and/or the Pain Perception Scale, or a child-orientated pain measure if appropriate

3   The short form of the McGill Pain Questionnaire (SF-MCQ)

4   The Hospital Anxiety and Depression Scale (the Leeds Scale, HADS) (see Fig. 13.1).

Physical examination

The assessment continues with the physical examination during which the clinician should watch for evidence of pain-related behavioural responses including wincing, groans or exclamations about pain, writhing, limping or avoidance of movements that the patient believes will cause or increase pain.

Points to observe during the examination

1   Always accept a patient's complaint as genuine, because failure to do so is likely to result in rejection of the clinician or, at best, a difficult interview. If the symptoms do not fit a pattern recognized as a specific disease or injury, for example angina, renal colic or a prolapsed lumbar intervertebral disc, the complaint is valid nevertheless and

Hospital Anxiety and Depression Scale (HADS)

nferNelson
understanding potential

Name:_____ Date: _____

FOLD HERE

Clinicians are aware that emotions play an important part in most illnesses. If your clinician knows about these feelings he or she will be able to help you more.

This questionnaire is designed to help your clinician to know how you feel. Read each item below and **underline the reply** which comes closest to how you have been feeling in the past week. Ignore the numbers printed at the edge of the questionnaire.

Don't take too long over your replies, your immediate reaction to each item will probably be more accurate than a long, thought-out response.

FOLD HERE

I feel tense or 'wound up'
Most of the time
A lot of the time
From time to time, occasionally
Not at all

I still enjoy the things I used to enjoy
Definitely as much
Not quite so much
Only a little
Hardly at all

I get a sort of frightened feeling as if something awful is about to happen
Very definitely and quite badly
Yes, but not too badly
A little, but it doesn't worry me
Not at all

I can laugh and see the funny side of things
As much as I always could
Not quite so much now
Definitely not so much now
Not at all

Worrying thoughts go through my mind
A great deal of the time
A lot of the time
Not too often
Very little

I feel cheerful
Never
Not often
Sometimes
Most of the time

I can sit at ease and feel relaxed
Definitely
Usually
Not often
Not at all

I feel as if I am slowed down
Nearly all the time
Very often
Sometimes
Not at all

I get a sort of frightened feeling like 'butterflies' in the stomach
Not at all
Occasionally
Quite often
Very often

I have lost interest in my appearance
Definitely
I don't take as much care as I should
I may not take quite as much care
I take just as much care as ever

I feel restless as if I have to be on the move
Very much indeed
Quite a lot
Not very much
Not at all

I look forward with enjoyment to things
As much as I ever did
Rather less than I used to
Definitely less than I used to
Hardly at all

I get sudden feelings of panic
Very often indeed
Quite often
Not very often
Not at all

I can enjoy a good book or radio or television programme
Often
Sometimes
Not often
Very seldom

Now check that you have answered all the questions

Fig 13.1 Hospital anxiety and depression scale (HADS). The Hospital Anxiety and Depression Scale is copyright to RP Snaith & AS Zigmoid. It is reproduced here by permission of the publishers, nferNelson Publishing Company, The Chiswick Centre, 414 Chiswick High Road, London W4 5TF. All rights reserved. nferNelson is a division of Granada Learning Ltd, part of Granada Inc.

represents a communication to the clinician about distress. That distress may well be psychologically determined, even though the symptom suggests a physical disorder.

2 Considerable information is obtained by observing the behaviour of patients with acute or chronic pain. Many

forms of pain give rise to specific behaviours, as in the case of an altered gait where there is a hip or knee injury. At times, behaviour may not seem appropriate because the patient's level of discomfort and disability is in excess of what is expected given the nature of the physical disorder. Alternatively, behaviour may be remarkably normal despite vehement complaints of severe and unremitting pain. In both situations the complaints and behaviour contrast with few or absent objective signs of a physical disorder. The behaviours may be helpful to the clinician because they indicate that psychological factors are likely to be playing a major part in the disorder. It is useful always to compare the behaviour shown by the patient during the interview with that exhibited at the time of physical examination – sometimes the differences are surprising and informative!

The interpretation of pain behaviours is described elsewhere, but a few key observations include watching the person dress or undress (by the clinician or a nurse), because this often reveals movements are possible that could not be demonstrated during the course of examination. It should be noted that if a person uses a walking stick it may not be serving as a true physical support, and is unnecessary therefore other than 'as a badge' of the patient's disabled status, or as a psychological 'crutch'. The presence of support collars, lumbar supports, or TENS machines, may well be quite appropriate; however, in some patients they are more symbolic than functional.

3   Patients with pain fall into three broad groups. First, there are those who have clear evidence of an acute or chronic physical cause for pain. Second are those who have a physical disorder, but show marked pain behaviour and emotional changes that are beyond what might normally be expected. In such circumstances failure of treatment, or failure to cope, with even modest levels of pain may be suspected. Third are those who do not have any evidence of a past or present physical condition that could account for their pain and disability. In this case there are two main possibilities to consider. The patient may have a somatoform disorder (see Ch. 12), or may be suffering from a mental disorder and, in particular, a depressive disorder. A third but less common cause might be malingering (deliberate falsification of symptoms) where compensation is being sought after an accident.

4   It is helpful when making an assessment, and especially in patients with chronic pain, to interview the closest relative, or a close friend, sometimes separately from the patient. Corroboration or otherwise of points in the patient's history should be sought, other aspects of family relationships will emerge, and the clinician has an opportunity to gain the relative's confidence. It is essential for the relatives to understand fully the diagnosis and aims of any management programme, because without their support and help such programmes usually fail.

Use pain terms correctly

In order to use the correct terms when defining different types of altered sensation, present at times in people with painful disorders, the following terms should be committed to memory.

Allodynia – pain elicited by a normally non-noxious stimulus such as light touch.

Anaesthesia dolorosa – the experience of pain in an area that is insensitive to normal levels of stimulation.

Analgesia – absence of pain in the presence of stimulation that normally gives rise to pain.

Dysaesthesia – an unpleasant abnormal sensation that may arise as a result of normal levels of stimulation, or spontaneously.

Hyperaesthesia – an increase in response or sensitivity to normal levels of stimulation.

Hypoaesthesia – decreased sensitivity to normal levels of stimulation.

Hyperalgesia – an increased response/sensitivity to stimuli that are normally painful, e.g. pinprick.

Hyperpathia – an increased reaction to a stimulus but with an increased threshold to it.

Hypoalgesia – decreased response to stimuli that are normally painful.

Paraesthesia – an abnormal sensation that may arise as a result of normal levels of stimulation, or spontaneously.

Principles of pain management

Making a diagnosis

The diagnosis of a painful condition is usually uncomplicated, but difficulty is often experienced when a sound physical basis for pain cannot be detected, or when the pain complaint and disability seem out of proportion to any underlying physical abnormality. Given that the assessment of the problem is based carefully upon the three elements of the history outlined (physical, emotional and social), and clues are sought from the clinical signs and behaviour shown at the time of physical examination, the clinician should not miss the diagnosis even of a condition that is driven by psychosocial factors. It may be helpful when such conditions are suspected to use the criteria from ICD 10 or DSM IV-R (see Ch. 13) in particular, because both provide a fixed framework of criteria for a diagnosis. Their use trains the clinicians to standardize their approach to the diagnosis of somatoform disorders and other mental disorders associated with pain.

Investigations

It is vital that the diagnosis of a pain condition is supported by the use of appropriate haematological, biochemical and radiological tests.

Discussion of the diagnosis with patients and their relatives

Improvements in clinical practice in recent years have led to greater involvement of patients and their relatives in the management of illness and disability. It is the duty of clinicians to practise and improve their communication skills and to interact in an effective manner (Box 13.1). A clear explanation of the nature of the condition with reasons for its causation should be given to the patient and the relatives. Patients should be given an uncomplicated and unambiguous explanation of the problem posed and the choices of treatment available. The clinician should not place responsibilities for the selection of treatments upon the patient, but should share the decision by guiding the patient towards the clinically preferred option. Potential difficulties and hazards of treatment, if any, should be discussed; however, this does not mean giving the patient every possible difficulty to consider, but only those that might reasonably be expected to occur or those with potentially serious consequences. Otherwise the patient may become unnecessarily anxious and may reject what is, in fact, quite rea-

Box 13.1

Communication skills

- Good clinician–patient communication is central to effective practice.

- Poor communication increases the risk of inaccurate diagnosis, patient dissatisfaction and failure to comply with treatments.

- There are several important factors influencing the effectiveness of clinician/patient communications and they include:

  — the physical setting/the interchange

  — non-verbal communications

  — verbal communication skills

  — the psychosocial context of the interaction including the effect of the clinician's personal characteristics upon the patient and vice versa.

- Effective clinical communication requires the ability to use the relevant skills flexibly in response to the needs of different patients.

From: Hypnosis and suggestion in the treatment of pain by Joseph Barber. Copyright (c)1996 by Joseph Barber. Used by permission of W.W. Norton & Company, Inc.

sonable treatment. The role of the clinician is that of the expert and a trained professional who guides and supports the patient.

Discussion of the diagnosis and plan for treatment with a close relative is advisable and the involvement of relatives in chronic pain management is especially important if the programme is to succeed. If relatives are not involved and are unaware of the clinical aims of the management team, especially where psychological methods of treatment are being used, they may unknowingly undermine the treatment programme.

Selection of treatment or management programme

Brief details of treatments for specific pain syndromes are dealt with in other chapters.

Evidence-based medicine

This text is not written to provide the reader with detailed information about evidence-based medicine, but being a good

Box 13.2

The basis for practising evidence-based medicine

- Forming clinical questions so that they can be answered.
- Searching for the best external evidence.
- Critically appraising the evidence for its validity and importance.
- Actually applying evidence in clinical practice.
- Self-evaluation as a practitioner of evidence-based medicine.

doctor means combining clinical expertise with the best available evidence from systematic research when making treatment decisions for individual patients (see Ch. 15). You should learn as much as possible from each clinical episode, and be up to date at all times with relevant literature – a life-long process. It is difficult, if not impossible, to remain fully informed in the many fields of medicine and to know all that is to be known about clinical aspects of pain management. Recently it has become possible to obtain clinically useful and up-to-date knowledge of growing numbers of randomized clinical trials of treatment through the process of meta-analyses and the publication of systematic reviews based upon them. This information is available through the Cochrane Library in York and the NHS Research and Development Centre for evidence-based medicine in Oxford. Those working in Oxford have a particular interest in clinical trials of treatments for pain and have an excellent website that publishes an electronic journal (Bandolier). This provides useful information about many aspects of evidence-based medicine.

The basis for the use of evidence-based medicine is summarized in Box 13.2.

Pain management services

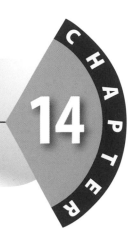

CHAPTER 14

Chapter objectives

After studying this chapter you should be able to:

1 Appreciate the role of acute pain management teams in education, delivery of care and planning of services.

2 Appreciate the role of chronic pain management services in delivery of care, education and planning of services.

3 Appreciate the problems of pain in the community and the role of primary care teams.

4 Appreciate the general philosophy of cancer pain management services and how these integrate with palliative care in hospitals, hospices and the community.

5 Understand that multidisciplinary team working is central to successful pain and symptom management.

6 Understand the need to integrate pain management services with primary care, other secondary care providers and palliative care.

Provision of acute pain services

It is now accepted that all acute services should provide appropriate pain management. Despite unprecedented interest in understanding pain mechanisms and pain management, a significant number of patients continue to experience unacceptable pain after surgery. Recent surveys show that there has been no apparent improvement since an early study in 1952. It is increasingly clear that the solution to the problems of postoperative pain management lies not so much in the development of new techniques but in developing an organization to exploit existing expertise. The major barriers to this are lack of organization and education, and are not usually related to the analgesic techniques themselves.

Acute pain teams

There is good evidence that analgesia in the acute setting is best delivered by specialist pain teams acting as support for staff, patients and carers. Acute pain teams (APTs) are there to provide education, advise about difficult acute pain problems, plan and monitor services and to take part in audit, research and risk management. The members of an APT include anaesthetists, surgeons, nurses, pharmacists and physiotherapists. Protocols encourage consistent standards of safe and effective care and should be used as a framework to individualize treatment. The concept of skilled pain therapists collaborating to provide improved postoperative analgesia within the framework of an organized acute pain service (APS) appears to be universally applicable. Acute pain service models have been described from the United States, the United Kingdom, Germany, Switzerland and Sweden. The means of providing satisfactory analgesia are already present in most hospitals. Careful planning and a multidisciplinary approach to pain management will ensure that resources are optimally utilized, and the quality of pain management is consistently maintained.

The provision of multidisciplinary APTs in acute UK hospitals performing adult inpatient surgery has been surveyed many times. There are well-demonstrated, positive associations between the presence of an APT and improvements in postoperative pain control. The presence of an APT is associated with more use of patient-controlled analgesia and epidural drug delivery, regular in-service training for nurses and junior doctors, written guidelines/protocols for management of postoperative pain, routine use of postoperative pain measurement systems and audit/research in relation to postoperative pain issues. APTs, in which nurses play a major role, have a pivotal influence in relation to not only postoperative analgesia but also wider service development. Since 1995, the number of hospitals offering inpatient surgery that are covered by an APT has risen.

Appropriate education is essential for all healthcare professionals involved in providing acute pain management. Staff education should be arranged to suit the local needs. Good pain assessment and documentation in clinical areas positively influences pain management. Acute pain is largely predictable and can largely be managed using guidelines for clinical practice. Standardization of analgesic protocols, equipment, monitoring, management of adverse events and clear documentation all improve the quality of pain management. Many professional bodies have produced guidelines for the management of acute pain. However, in many countries the provision of such services is variable and inconsistent. There is evidence that the provision of an acute pain service results in a significant improvement in acute postoperative pain management and a reduction in complications such as emesis. It may also facilitate rehabilitation and reduce hospital stay. Patient and carer education is vital, and support is best delivered before surgery wherever possible, although in pain from trauma this is not practical. Patients may be given booklets or shown short videos about aspects of pain control.

Acute pain after day-case surgery

Day-case surgery is of great value to patients and the health service. It enables many more patients to be treated properly, and faster than before. Newer, less invasive, operative techniques will allow many more procedures to be carried out. There are many elements to successful day-case surgery, for example the effectiveness of the control of pain after the operation, and the effectiveness of measures to minimize postoperative nausea and vomiting. Day surgery is not without complications, with 26% of patients experiencing notable degrees of pain, 23% having minor medical problems after discharge and 8% of respondents having to reattend hospital with problems relating to their original operations. Unplanned hospital readmission is a measure of quality of care in the setting of day-case surgery; pain and emesis are common causes of this problem. The increasing demand to reduce waiting lists for elective surgery by performing more day-case operations means that pain control is especially important. There is a lack of knowledge about patients' experiences of postoperative pain at home.

Surveys show that, despite modern anaesthesia and surgery, about a fifth of patients have severe pain immediately following day-case surgery. The majority of patients leave day-case wards in pain and have pain at some time between 2 and 4 days' postoperatively. Severe levels of pain following discharge from hospital are a concern for a fifth of patients. Day-case staff do not always ask patients whether they are in pain, when it is known that communication with patients is vital in the delivery of optimal care. In day surgery, the availability of a unified and reliable measure of pain that can address its sensory component, such as the VAS, will provide more reliable information about the pain experience and hence improve its overall management. Quality of home recovery may be improved by: wider use of perioperative analgesia, systematic prescription of take-home analgesia, designation of a hospital practitioner for advice and closer collaboration with general practitioners. More support and more information are needed to manage patients' pain effectively whilst in the day-case wards and also following discharge, at home. Due to the importance of quality assurance and cost containment in healthcare, eliciting patients' preferences for postoperative outcomes may be a more economical and reliable method of assessing quality. Avoidance of postoperative pain and nausea and vomiting is a major priority for day-case patients. Anaesthetists should take patients' preferences into consideration when developing guidelines and planning anaesthetic care.

Acute pain in children

Acute pain control in paediatrics is a particular problem. Behavioural changes have been reported in children after surgery, and it has been concluded that postoperative pain significantly affects their occurrence. Much pain in children can be well managed if recommendations about the logical use of analgesic drugs are followed, for example appropriate drug doses, given by appropriate routes at set times rather than when pain has occurred and become moderate/severe. The provision and organization of paediatric acute pain services are often poor. Recent surveys in the UK have shown, for example, that despite the widespread use of epidural analgesia in children its place in paediatric pain management has not been clearly established. There was little consensus regarding drugs and drug combinations used for epidural analgesia. One-third of UK paediatric centres did not audit their epidural practice, and of those that did the reported incidences of side effects showed wide variation. Important differences in practice were also identified in the areas of patient selection, informed consent, the use of epidural test doses, drug delivery systems, monitoring and the management of side effects. Twelve per cent of UK specialist paediatric hospitals did not have an acute pain team and elsewhere the provision was often limited to staff with few or no specialist skills. Inconsistencies are likely to be related to the poor evidence base available to guide clinical decision making and the lack of a specialized paediatric acute pain service in some centres. Clinical support for paediatric pain control should be more widely available.

Pain control in children after day-case surgery is a particular challenge. Day-case surgery is designed to keep children within their families. Day-case surgery involves a considerable amount of stress not only for the children who undergo surgery but also for their parents. The main factors influencing the amount of stress experienced by parents are feelings of insufficient preparation and problems with postoperative pain at home. Parents of children having day-case surgery must be adequately informed and supported. A telephone call following day-case surgery appears to give parents effective support.

Chronic pain management services

John Bonica, an American anaesthetist and founder of the International Association for the Study of Pain pioneered the concept of multidisciplinary clinics for patients with persistent pain in the 1950s. However, it took until the 1970s before pain management clinics became more widely established. The principle of simultaneous treatment of physical, psychological and social aspects of pain is now accepted. Anaesthetists were involved in setting up the early pain services, using nerve-blocking skills that they had learned for anaesthesia and acute pain. Although good pain management is now far more than simple nerve blocks, many anaesthetists worldwide have specialized in pain management. Pain management needs inter-disciplinary cooperation between healthcare professionals. Pain management uses a multidisciplinary team approach that matches therapy to the individual patient. Various healthcare professionals (e.g. nurse specialists, physiotherapists, clinical psychologists, occupational therapists and pharmacists) make an important contribution to pain management. Efficient and effective pain management requires close links between

Box 14.1

Functions of a chronic pain management service

- Multimodal management of pain that is resistant to treatment.
- Management of psychological distress.
- Management of behavioural problems.
- Reduction of disability.
- Restoration of function.
- Optimization of medication.
- Recognition of social, family and occupational issues.
- Liaison with other healthcare professionals in primary and secondary care.
- Education for healthcare professionals.
- Audit and evaluation of pain management.
- Advising providers about the needs of patients with persistent pain and their carers.
- Research into the epidemiology, causes and management of pain.

medical specialties (e.g. surgery, medicine, rheumatology, gastroenterology, neurology, elderly medicine, rehabilitation medicine, occupational health, oncology, palliative medicine, psychiatry, addiction medicine, paediatrics and primary care).

A chronic pain management service has many functions (Box 14.1). There needs to be provision of basic chronic pain management services within all secondary care services. There should be selective provision of specialist pain management services on a regional basis. All pain management teams should provide both hospital and community care to patients with a wide range of different conditions. Close cooperation with primary care teams is essential. There must be special provision for vulnerable and potentially disadvantaged groups such as older people, children, people with learning difficulties and patients from diverse ethnic backgrounds whose first language may not be the country's native language. Patients with impaired hearing or vision should have their special needs addressed. Particular difficulties may be encountered with problem drug users, prisoners and survivors of torture. Patients from all these groups need, and should have, access to appropriate pain management services.

Pain services provide treatments for pain, but just as importantly, have an educational role for patients and their carers. It is important that patients understand the difference between acute and chronic pain and have any misconceptions about the meaning of pain explained. Much of the work of chronic pain services is to reduce disability and improve function by helping patients overcome their fears about what pain means. As well as explaining pain mechanisms and treatment strategies to patients, written information should be available explaining the treatments available in the pain management unit in a way that is readily understandable. This must cater for all patients, including those with special requirements. Patients must be able to make an informed decision about the pain management treatments that they choose.

Pain in the community and the role of primary care teams

Pain is the commonest reason that patients present for medical attention; for example headache and back pain are amongst the most frequent reasons that patients consult their general practitioner. It is important that the primary care team provides the appropriate diagnostic and triage service for those with acute or new pain problems. These patients should be given analgesia and then investigated and, if necessary, referred to secondary care services.

Pain in the elderly is common and it is essential that physicians and other healthcare professionals looking after residents in long-term care facilities be proficient in the recognition, assessment and treatment of chronic pain. A holistic approach to the physical, emotional, social and spiritual components of a resident's total pain and distress must be integrated into the palliative aspects of long-term care medicine. Furthermore, all practitioners must recognize and effectively manage the acute pain, breakthrough pain and incident pain that are frequently superimposed on a resident's chronic pain.

Chronic pain is prevalent and therefore much of its management occurs in the community rather than in specialist units. About two-thirds of chronic pain seen in primary care is musculoskeletal. Primary care faces the challenge of reducing the proportion of patients continuing with musculoskeletal pain beyond the acute phase. There is a strong association between pain-related disability and greater use of healthcare services. Initial pain intensity, behavioural problems and previous pain episodes are factors predictive of chronicity. Studies have shown that disabling low back pain persisted in one-third of participants after consultation with the general practitioner. It was more common with increasing age, among those with a history of low back pain and in women. Persistence of symptoms was associated with 'premorbid' factors (high levels of psychological distress, poor self-rated health, low levels of physical activity, smoking, dissatisfaction with employment) and factors related to the episode of low back pain (duration of symptoms, pain radiating to the leg, widespread pain and restriction in spinal mobility). Patients at high risk of chronic pain should be identified and managed at an early stage. Appropriate analgesic prescribing, referral for simple physical treatments (e.g. spinal manipulation) and positive reinforcement to increase activity are often effective strategies that can easily take place in a community setting. Inappropriate referral to and long waiting times for orthopaedic opinions in patients without significant clinical indicators of a surgical lesion should be avoided. Similarly, radiological investigations are needed only in those with back pain who fulfil certain criteria and should be avoided in others. Their use is costly, often delays active management and reinforces the patient's belief that there are serious structural problems. The Royal College of General Practitioners in the UK has developed guidelines for the management of acute back pain. Simple changes in practice can affect outcomes; for example a change from the traditional prescription of bed rest for acute back pain to positive advice about staying active within primary care could improve clinical outcomes and reduce the personal and social impact of back pain.

Primary care teams need to develop integrated and multi-professional care pathways for management of common chronic pain problems. Patients can be categorized according to their level of disability based on ratings of pain intensity, activity interference, emotional distress, perceived support and work disability. Then treatment algorithms can be developed for patients considered to have moderate or high disability. Algorithms and recommendations for the use of drugs are important in improving consistency of chronic pain management in primary care (e.g. recommendations for the use of opioids in persistent non-cancer pain). There is increased community use of non-pharmacological techniques such as acupuncture, massage and relaxation. These treatments need to be evidence based and applied in a consistent manner.

Nurse-led chronic pain clinics have been developed in primary care. These often use structured questionnaires and interviews, and treatment and interventions are based on local guidelines. The use of such services can reduce waiting times and result in more appropriate and timely referrals to secondary care. Integrating a comprehensive approach to pain with local specialist pain services gives the primary care physician and patient the greatest chance for success.

Cancer pain management services

The worldwide incidence of cancer has increased and, in spite of major therapeutic advances, many tumours remain incurable. Cancer pain is a significant problem for millions of people and their carers. Adequate control of this pain can improve quality of life and is an essential part of palliation. A team of healthcare professionals should provide physical, psychosocial and spiritual support.

In patients with cancer, pain management is part of the broader therapeutic endeavour of palliative care that is both a philosophy of care and an organized highly structured system for delivering care. Its goal is to prevent and relieve suffering and support the best possible quality of life for patients and their families, regardless of the stage of the disease or the need for other therapies. Palliative care expands traditional disease-model medical treatments and involves enhancing quality of life for the patient and family, optimizing function, helping with decision making and providing opportunities for personal growth. It can occur alongside life-prolonging care, or as the focus of care. It involves a team of healthcare professionals who provide continuing management including control of pain and symptoms, maintenance of function, psychosocial and spiritual support for the patient and family, and comprehensive care at the end of life.

The multiprofessional team is the foundation of good palliative care. It is important to consider different perspectives regarding the patient and their pain and to explore all methods of pain management (e.g. physical as well as drug-related therapies). The team must address psychological, social and spiritual aspects of care that will have a bearing on patients' physical pain. Using a physical technique to manage pain that has significant non-physical elements will result in disappointment. A careful assessment at the outset will avoid the situation where a patient is subjected to an invasive procedure with little chance of benefit. Patient choice is paramount to all decision making in palliative care and pain management. Where appropriate and at the patient's request, the family/carers should be included in discussions. For patients to make an informed choice, they must be fully apprised of all the options by an experienced professional who can discuss the details of any proposed procedure, the likely outcomes and possible adverse effects.

Information should also be given about the nature of after-care required and arrangements needed to continue care in the home. In many countries there are well developed home care teams that are coordinated within the community by palliative medicine units in partnership with primary care teams. These are supported by specialist palliative care nurses and other healthcare professionals (e.g. pharmacists, physiotherapists, social workers and occupational therapists). It is a fundamental principle that most patients want to die at home, so services should be designed to accommodate this, including good pain management. However, the place of death of cancer patients has become an important theme in UK cancer and palliative care policy. Studies have now revealed that there is a much stronger preference for deaths in a hospice than had been anticipated, leading to the need to reassess delivery of palliative care services in the community.

Management of acute pain

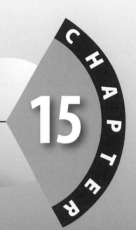

15

CHAPTER

Chapter objectives

After studying this chapter you should be able to:

1 Understand the definition of acute pain and recognize situations where acute pain may occur.

2 Understand the adverse physical and psychological effects of acute pain.

3 Understand that acute pain may become chronic.

4 Understand the concept of comparing analgesics by numbers needed to treat (NNT).

5 Know about systemic analgesics for acute pain management.

6 Know about local, regional and spinal analgesia for acute pain management.

7 Understand the use of different routes of drug administration.

8 Understand the role of non-pharmacological interventions for acute pain.

The nature of acute pain

Acute pain is pain of recent onset and probable limited duration; it usually has an identifiable and causal relationship to injury or disease. There are many causes for acute pain (Table 15.1).

Adverse effects of acute pain

Acute pain produces adverse physiological and psychological effects. The magnitude of the injury response depends on the nature and extent of the trauma; it may include inflammation, hypercoagualbility, catabolism, increased sympathetic nervous activity, hormonal changes and immune suppression (Fig. 15.1).

Pain can:

- Restrict breathing
- Prevent coughing
- Cause hypoxaemia, atelectasis and chest infection
- Increase in sympathetic output causing tachycardia, hypertension and increased myocardial oxygen requirement
- Cause myocardial ischaemia especially in those with other cardiovascular risk factors
- Result in reduced gastrointestinal function and ileus.

Appropriate pain management can modify the effects of tissue injury; however, an effect of analgesia on mortality has never been shown conclusively.

Table 15.1 Examples of causes of acute pain

Cause	Examples
Trauma	Fractures, burns, nerve injury
Pregnancy and childbirth	Back pain, labour
Surgery	Thoracotomy, laparotomy
Procedures	Wound drainage, pressure sore care
Medical conditions	Dental pain, appendicitis, pancreatitis, sickle cell crisis, migraine, acute low back pain, renal colic
Cancer	Spinal cord compression, pathological fractures
Infection	Acute herpes zoster, encephalitis

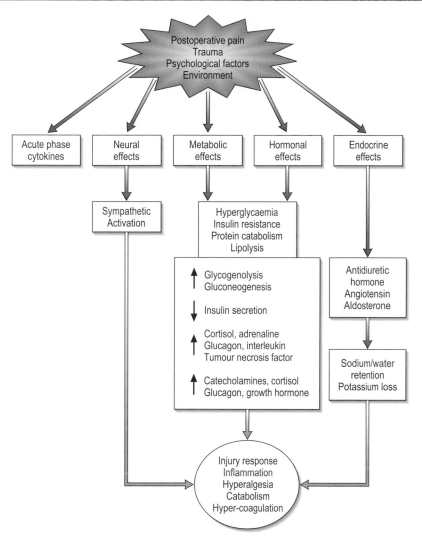

Fig 15.1 The injury response.

Psychosocial factors contribute to the acute pain experience. Preoperative anxiety or depression is associated with increased postoperative pain. Mood can affect the use of techniques such as patient-controlled analgesia (PCA), where the patient self-administers analgesics. Anxious or depressed patients make more PCA demands and have less good quality analgesia. Therefore poor pain relief may cause sleep disturbance, anxiety and other adverse psychological effects.

Transition from acute to chronic pain

Acute and chronic pain may represent a continuum rather than distinct entities. Patients often relate a chronic pain condition to an acute incident; for example postoperative, post-traumatic, acute back pain and acute herpes zoster can all lead to chronic pain. There are a number of risk factors for development of chronic pain after surgery, for example severe pain before surgery, multiple surgeries, intraoperative nerve damage, limb amputation and pre-existing mood problems. Acute herpes zoster is more likely to develop into postherpetic neuralgia if the initial pain is severe. Specific early analgesia may reduce the likelihood of development of persistent pain. Preventative analgesia is therefore important.

Assessment and comparison of analgesic techniques

The number needed to treat (NNT) for one patient to achieve at least 50% pain relief is a useful way of expressing efficacy and comparing analgesics. The most effective treatments have an NNT of just over 2. This means that for every two patients who receive the drug one patient will get at least 50% relief because of treatment. A similar concept is NNH (number needed to harm) when looking at adverse events.

Systemic analgesics

The route of administration is as important as the choice of drug:

- If possible, the oral route should be used for mild to moderate pain. Many simple analgesic and adjuvant drugs are well absorbed after oral dosing.

- It is important to use immediate release preparations for acute pain.

- Transdermal or modified release drugs are not useful in acute pain because dose adjustment and titration are too slow.

- Other routes may be needed if the patient cannot swallow and absorb or is nil by mouth for other reasons.

- In each person, there is a minimum effective analgesic blood concentration (MEAC) that is needed to achieve pain relief. If a 4-hourly intramuscular opioid-dosing regimen is used, plasma concentration exceeds the MEAC for only 35% of the time. To sustain stable plasma concentrations it is logical and more controllable to give opioids intravenously rather than as intermittent intramuscular boluses. Peak analgesia occurs 10–20 minutes after administration of intravenous morphine. This must be preceded by a loading dose to achieve MEAC that would otherwise take four to six times the elimination half-life of the drug. Therefore, it is important to use such a loading dose at the beginning of treatment or if analgesia is lost.

- A fourfold difference in MEAC is often reported in clinical studies where opioids are given intravenously, reflecting individual differences in drug requirements.

- The use of injectable formulations alone does not guarantee better analgesia. Absorption is reliable, but sometimes quite slow, following intramuscular opioids, for example peak analgesia is not achieved until 60–90 minutes after intramuscular morphine injection and is delayed in shock.

- Inhalation of nitrous oxide in oxygen or transmucosal oral fentanyl may be useful for transient, severe pain and to provide analgesia for procedures.

- Sublingual administration of opioids reduces 'first pass' metabolism; however, the drug must be very lipid soluble and potent to be given by this route (e.g. buprenorphine).

- Rectal administration produces variable absorption; morphine and oxycodone have been used in this way, but there is a large variation within and between subjects.

Simple analgesics

Indications Paracetamol is a good simple analgesic and antipyretic. It is effective when given alone for mild pain, and it can be used in combination with weak (e.g. codeine) or strong (e.g. oxycodone) opioids for moderate pain.

Pharmacology Its mechanism of action is not clear, but it probably acts by inhibiting central cyclo-oxygenase 2 and 3 type receptors and via descending 5-HT pathways.

It is rapidly absorbed from the small intestine after oral administration. The rectal route can also be used. A parenteral formulation is available. The antipyretic dose is lower than the analgesic dose. Attention is needed to dosing; in adults the maximum daily oral dose is 4 g. However, children are often underdosed because the dose is given on an age-contingent basis, rather than using the child's weight to calculate the requirement (see below). The rectal route produces unreliable absorption, and 1 g every 6 hours may be subtherapeutic for some adults. The rectal route should be used only if the patient cannot take or absorb oral medication. Paracetamol 1g has an NNT of nearly 5; combination of paracetamol with other drugs

Table 15.2 Oral analgesic efficacy (NNTs) for 50% pain relief over 4–6 hours: single dose studies in patients with acute moderate to severe pain

Analgesic	Dose (mg)	NNT
Valdecoxib	20	1.7
Diclofenac	100	1.9
Paracetamol/codeine	1000/60	2.2
Parecoxib*	40	2.2
Diclofenac	50	2.3
Ibuprofen	600	2.4
Ibuprofen	400	2.4
Ketorolac	10	2.6
Ibuprofen	200	2.7
Diclofenac	25	2.8
Pethidine*	100	2.9
Morphine*	10	2.9
Parecoxib*	20	3.0
Paracetamol	500	3.5
Paracetamol	1000	3.8
Paracetamol/codeine	600–650/60	4.2
Aspirin	600–650	4.4
Celecoxib	200	4.5
Paracetamol	600–650	4.6
Tramadol	100	4.8
Tramadol	50	8.3
Codeine	60	16.7

* Parenteral.

improves the NNT (Table 15.2). Adverse effects: Paracetamol does not affect peripheral cyclo-oxygenase receptors, so it has fewer side effects than anti-inflammatory agents. It does not lead to bleeding; it can be used in asthmatics or those at risk of peptic ulcers. It should be avoided in patients with active liver disease.

Non-steroidal anti-inflammatory drugs (NSAIDs) and cyclo-oxygenase 2 (COX-2) inhibitors

Indications These are effective analgesic and anti-inflammatory drugs in many acute pains. They may be more effective when given for more than a few days. They are useful alone for mild to moderate pain. They are also used in combination with paracetamol for mild to moderate pain and with strong opioids for severe pain. When they are given with opioids after surgery, they reduce the opioid requirement by about 25–50%.

Pharmacology Prostaglandins are produced by prostaglandin endoperoxide synthase that involves COX sites. COX-1 enzymes regulate some of the physiological functions, for example gut protection, maintaining renal function in stress, bronchodilatation and platelet function. They also have important effects on the reproductive and central nervous systems. Pain, inflammation and tissue damage lead to the production of COX-2 enzymes; these are also normally present in the lung, kidney, ovary and testis. NSAIDs inhibit COX-1 and -2 enzymes non-specifically.

Different formulations can be given orally, rectally, topically or parenterally. There is no evidence that using the rectal route leads to better analgesia or reduces side effects; the only reason to use this route is if the patient cannot take oral drugs. Topical NSAIDs are effective and they may be used for mild acute musculoskeletal pains.

Adverse effects NSAIDs and COX-2 inhibitors have some common side effects, e.g. on renal function, but there are differences, e.g. gastrointestinal effects.

Salicylates   *Indications* They are used alone in mild to moderate pain and in combination with stronger drugs in more severe pain. They may be used in low dose for their antiplatelet activity.

Pharmacology These are the oldest class of NSAIDs. Aspirin has a central and peripheral analgesic and antipyretic effect after a single dose; about 3.6 g aspirin daily is needed for anti-inflammatory action.

Adverse effects These are common, for example the gastric irritation and tinnitus that occur at high doses and limit its usefulness. Aspirin is a particular problem because it has an irreversible effect for the life of the platelet, even after a single dose. Enteric-coated aspirin reduces occult gastrointestinal bleeding; however, it has not been shown to affect the incidence of serious gastrointestinal effects. Aspirin causes bronchospasm in 10–15% of patients with asthma, chronic rhinitis and nasal polyps. Aspirin must be avoided in children because of the risk of potentially fatal Reyes syndrome.

Other oral NSAIDs

Indications These do very well in the single dose postoperative comparisons of NNT (Table 15.2).

Pharmacology Pharmacokinetic differences in these drugs do not explain the individual variation seen in response to NSAIDs and COX-2 inhibitors. Plasma half-life does not reflect the duration of analgesia that is sometimes shorter or longer than expected.

Adverse effects NSAIDs produce significant adverse effects, for example peptic ulceration, bleeding, renal impairment, bronchospasm, fluid retention with cardiac compromise and some cognitive effects; many of these are commoner in the elderly. These problems can occur in the acute setting; however, they are more likely with long-term use. Renal prostaglandins maintain renal blood flow in stress situations such as hypovolaemia and renal impairment. Therefore, in the perioperative or trauma situation, even brief use of NSAIDs can cause renal problems in susceptible patients, for example the elderly, those in shock or with pre-existing renal disease and patients taking other drugs with adverse renal effects (e.g. gentamicin or ACE inhibitors). NSAIDs, even in single dose, inhibit platelet function and can increase bleeding after surgery. This problem is increased by other factors that cause bleeding, for example bleeding diathesis, shock and anticoagulant drugs. Prostaglandins are produced in the gut to protect the mucosa. Even short-term NSAID use can cause peptic ulceration and bleeding. The risks are increased with high doses and prolonged use in those with a history of ulcers, smokers, those on steroids or anticoagulants, and in the elderly.

COX-2 inhibitors

Indications These drugs have been used in patients who are at risk from the gastrointestinal and antiplatelet effects of NSAIDs.

Pharmacology These drugs specifically inhibit COX-2 (e.g. meloxicam, celecoxib, etoricoxib, valdecoxib and parecoxib); these agents vary in their selectivity for COX-2. These are available as oral formulations apart from parecoxib, which is a prodrug of valdecoxib that can be given parenterally.

Adverse effects These drugs are as effective as NSAIDs for acute pain (Table 15.2), but have fewer gut side effects and they are not antiplatelet. Platelets only produce COX-1, so the more selective the COX-2 inhibitor the less effect it has on bleeding. The perioperative use of COX-2 inhibitors causes less surgical bleeding than when NSAIDs are used. Their renal effects are similar to NSAIDs, so the same caution is needed. There is controversy about whether COX-2 drugs can promote thrombosis, and this issue remains to be clarified. There is some evidence for increased risk of cerebrovascular and cardiovascular adverse events when COX-2 agents are used and concerns about their use have resulted in the withdrawal of some of these drugs.

Opioids

Indications Moderate to severe acute pain requires opioids.

Pharmacology Opioids are agonists at endogenous receptors, such as μ, κ, and δ sites, in the periphery, spinal cord and brain. Some opioids display differential receptor activity; the clinical relevance of this is not clear.

- Opioids include all drugs, naturally occurring and synthetic, that bind to opioid receptors and exert an effect.

- Opiates are drugs that are structurally related to opium alkaloids.

- Narcotic is largely a historical term, and should be abandoned, as it merely alludes to the sedative properties of most opioids.

- Opioid agonists bind to receptors and exert effects that increase with increasing dose. Agonists may bind to the same receptor, but have different efficacies, for example morphine is more efficacious than codeine.

- Partial agonists bind to a receptor and exert an effect that increases with increasing dose until it reaches a plateau (e.g. buprenorphine).

- Antagonists bind to a receptor and have no effect (e.g. naloxone).

- Agonist–antagonists act as agonists at one receptor subtype, and antagonists at a different population of receptors.

  Some aspects of opioid pharmacology that are observed in the laboratory do not produce the predicted effects in the clinical setting, for example partial agonists may have a ceiling effect for analgesia where increasing dose does not lead to improved pain relief, but in clinical situations this is not usually a problem. There is no clinical interaction between morphine and buprenorphine, if the drugs are given together. Less than 1% of the opioid receptors need to be occupied to produce analgesia after 10 mg morphine is administered. If an equipotent dose of buprenorphine is given, about 6% opioid receptor occupancy is needed to produce analgesia. Therefore, an excess of receptors are available in normal circumstances, and buprenorphine does not reverse the effect of morphine.

Opioids are classified as weak (e.g. codeine) or strong (e.g. morphine) (Table 15.3). The distinction between these groups is not always clear and may depend on the dose. The term 'weak opioid' should not encourage lack of caution in prescribing. Analgesia is similar for all full agonist opioids if equipotent doses are used. There is huge variation in patients' responses to opioids, so that doses should be individualized and analgesia balanced against adverse effects. If a patient does not respond to a particular opioid or experiences limiting side effects, then it is reasonable to try a different opioid (opioid rotation or switching).

Opioids are metabolized in the liver to active and inactive products; many metabolites are conjugated with glucuronic acid and excreted renally, so care is needed when administering opioids to patients with poor renal function. Total body clearance is a measure of the efficiency of drug elimination and is affected by changes in hepatic perfusion. If plasma concentrations in excess of the minimum effective analgesic concentration are to be maintained, then drugs such as fentanyl that have a high clearance need to be given more frequently than those with a low clearance such as methadone, which tends to accumulate. There is no simple relationship between blood opioid concentrations, clearance and analgesia.

Adverse effects Opioids produce similar dose-related side effects when they are given in equipotent doses. There is no need to withhold opioids from patients with pain because of fears about dependence or tolerance either short or long term. If the pain remains constant, patients may be maintained on the same dose of an opioid for many months. Side effects include the following:

- Centrally mediated ventilatory depression occurs after opioid administration; this is not clinically important when opioids are titrated against opioid-sensitive pain. It is best detected by sedation rather than ventilatory rate. Therefore, it is important that patients who have opioids after surgery

Table 15.3 Opioid formulations[a]

Approved name	Formulations
Weak opioids	
Codeine	Oral
Dextropropoxyphene[b]	Oral
Dihydrocodeine	Oral
(DF118Forte, DHC Continus)	
Meptazinol	Oral
(Meptid)	
Tramadol[c]	Oral, parenteral
(Zydol, Zamadol)	
Strong opioids	
Alfentanil, remifentanil	Parenteral
Buprenorphine	Sublingual
(Temgesic, Transtec, BuTrans)	Transdermal, parenteral
Dextromoramide[b]	Oral
(Palfium)	
Diamorphine (heroin)	Oral, parenteral
Dipipanone[b]	Oral
(Diconal)	
Fentanyl	Transmucosal, oral
(Durogesic, Actiq)	Transdermal, parenteral
Hydromorphone	Oral, parenteral
(Palladone, Palladone SR)	
Methadone	Oral
Morphine (Oramorph, Sevredol, MST Continus, MXL, Zomorph)	Oral, parenteral
Oxycodone	Oral
(OxyNorm, OxyContin)	
Pentazocine[b]	Oral, parenteral
Pethidine[b]	Oral, parenteral
Tramadol[c]	Oral, parenteral
(Zydol, Zamadol)	

[a] Refer to *British National Formulary* for up-to-date dosage recommendations in adults and to specific paediatric formularies for children. Oral formulations may be immediate or modified release.

[b] Other drugs have superseded these agents and their use should be avoided.

[c] Tramadol may behave as a strong or a weak opioid depending on the dose used.

Some of the opioids are presented with paracetamol as compound analgesic preparations, e.g. co-codamol, Kapake, Solpadol, Tylex, co-dydramol, co-proxamol.

or trauma have supplementary oxygen and oxygen saturation monitoring.

- Opioid-related emesis is very common; it improves after a few days of opioid administration. Emesis following opioids is caused by stimulation of the chemoreceptor trigger zone, and is worse in ambulant patients. Opioid-induced nausea and vomiting should be treated by centrally acting drugs such as cyclizine, rather than those acting peripherally such as metoclopramide or domperidone.

- Dysphoria can occur with any opioid; the incidence with morphine is about 2–4%. It may be more of a problem with other opioids (e.g. nalbuphine).

- Opioid-induced itching is common and may be treated with low doses of naloxone, naltrexone, nalbuphine and ondansetron.

- Most opioids cause spasm of smooth muscle. Equianalgesic doses of fentanyl, pethidine and morphine increase the pressure in the common bile duct by 99, 61 and 53% respectively. Therefore, there is no advantage in choosing a particular opioid for biliary or renal colic.

- Constipation is a serious problem for patients taking opioids. Regular review of bowel function is important to prevent constipation becoming difficult to manage. A combination of stimulant and softening aperients should be prescribed for all patients who are taking opioids long term. It should be treated because it often results in patients being unable to tolerate opioids. Constipation is an important problem that persists and should be managed with aperients including drugs that increase bowel motility and stool softeners.

Codeine is a prodrug of morphine. About 2–10% of the dose given is metabolized to morphine; however, 10% of people do not have the enzyme necessary to do this, and so codeine is completely ineffective for them. It is not a good analgesic and produces significant side effects.

Dextropropoxyphene is often used in combination with paracetamol; it does not improve the analgesia and has side effects. It is dangerous in overdose. Its use should be avoided.

Dihydrocodeine is a useful weak opioid, but like all drugs of this class it is constipating.

Tramadol is different to the other opioids in that it has two mechanisms of action; it is an opioid agonist and a 5-TH and norepinephrine reuptake inhibitor. It has less respiratory depressant effects than the other opioids when given in equipotent dose. It has a similar incidence of emesis, but less effect on gut motility, so constipation is less common.

Morphine is the standard strong opioid used for moderate to severe pain; all other opioids are usually compared with it. It is available as an oral immediate release formulation. It is a hydrophilic and so is less well absorbed after oral dosing than some other opioids. There is large individual variation in the oral bioavailabilty of morphine (15–64%); therefore, titration of the dose against pain is essential. Less lipid-soluble opioids such as morphine are subject to hepatic 'first pass' metabolism. It is metabolized to morphine-3-glucuronide that is not analgesic and morphine-6-glucuronide that has analgesic properties. The oral parenteral ratio for morphine in patients receiving regular doses is about 3 : 1, less than the 6 : 1 ratio found in single dose studies, because of the contribution of active morphine metabolites. The accumulation of metabolites may lead to toxicity in patients with renal failure, so there are better opioids than morphine in this situation.

Fentanyl is a potent opioid that was largely confined to perioperative anaesthesia practice, but its rapid onset and potency has led to it being increasingly used for other acute pains.

Alfentanil and remifentanil are potent, short-acting opioids that are largely confined to anaesthesia and intensive care use.

Hydromorphone and oxycodone are both useful in the acute pain setting; there is little evidence for a difference in efficacy and side effects from morphine if equipotent doses are used.

Methadone has excellent oral bioavailability; it is potent and has a long duration of action. Its use in acute pain is limited and it may accumulate in hepatorenal failure.

Pethidine used to be used for patients with hepatobiliary and renal colic because it was believed to cause less smooth muscle spasm than morphine. In fact, it is no better than morphine, and has significant disadvantages such as production of toxic metabolites and addictive potential; its use should be avoided.

Adjuvant analgesics

A variety of drugs can be used to supplement simple analgesics, NSAIDs, COX-2 inhibitors and opioids (for more detailed pharmacology see Ch. 16).

Antidepressants and anticonvulsants

Antidepressants are commonly used, especially tricyclics. They are effective in the management of chronic neuropathic pain, but there is little data on their use in the acute situation. The use of antidepressants for acute pain may lead to a reduction in chronic pain after breast surgery or acute herpes zoster. Similarly, although there is good data to support the use of anticonvulsant drugs for chronic neuropathic pain, there is little evidence for their use in the acute pain situation.

It may be useful to treat patients at great risk of neuropathic pain with prophylactic antidepressants or anticonvulsants, but the dose should be low and any potential advantages must be balanced against adverse effects. Further good clinical trials are needed to support such practice.

Alpha₂ agonists Drugs of this type (e.g. clonidine and dexmedetomidine) can be used to reduce opioid requirements after surgery. Side effects are common with high doses, for example sedation and hypotension, and this may limit their use.

Inhalational analgesics

Nitrous oxide is a good analgesic with few side effects that can be given with oxygen as a 50 : 50 mixture for acute pain. It is commonly used in labour, trauma situations and for procedural pain, for example dental surgery, wound or burn care and dressing changes. When it is inhaled, it reaches analgesic concentrations in the brain within a few minutes. It wears off quickly and completely when inhalation ceases. It is more diffusible than nitrogen and oxygen, and so it will rapidly expand into air-filled spaces. It must not be used in patients with pneumothorax, pneumocephalus, middle ear obstruction, bowel obstruction and gas embolism, or after recent retinal surgery.

Long-term use may lead to bone marrow and neurological problems, but this is not relevant in the acute, single use situation.

Ketamine

Indications It can be used intravenously and intramuscularly as an anaesthetic for surgery and procedural pain, for example burns dressings. It is particularly useful in field and conflict situations and when there are mass casualties; for example it can be given intramuscularly to allow amputation during extrication from vehicles. It can also be used at subanaesthetic dosage for its analgesic properties.

Pharmacology Ketamine is an antagonist at *N*-methyl-D-aspartate (NMDA) receptors that mediate nociception. It is a potent analgesic and dissociative anaesthetic agent. It can be given orally, but there is little good evidence for efficacy. Its metabolite norketamine probably has an analgesic effect when this route is used. There is no place for its oral use in acute pain. Ketamine has an opioid-sparing effect and may be helpful in opioid-resistant pain.

Adverse effects Ketamine had side effects including tachycardia, hypertension, increasing intracranial pressure and unpleasant psychomimetic effects. It should not be used after head injury and care is needed with patients who have cardiovascular problems.

Patient-controlled analgesia

Patient-controlled analgesia (PCA) systems allow patients to regulate their own pain relief by delivering a dose of intravenous opioid on demand by the use of a button. Patients prefer this system to conventional parenteral regimens. The risk of ventilatory depression on general wards is increased by the use of continuous opioid infusions rather then PCA.

The use of a background infusion, the size of the bolus and the time during which no further demands will be met (lockout time) can all be varied. The optimum bolus dose in adults seems to be 1 mg for morphine and 40 µg for fentanyl, but bolus doses may need adjusting. The lockout interval is usually set between 5 and 12 minutes; this may also need review.

Intravenous PCA provides better analgesia than intravenous infusion, intramuscular and subcutaneous opioid regimens. PCA use may decrease the risk of pulmonary complications after surgery. Its use does not reduce opioid consumption, opioid side effects or improve the time to discharge from hospital. It is possible that the outcomes after PCA would be improved if prescriptions were more individualized. Many factors may increase the number of failed demands as well as pain, for example anxiety or failure to understand how the system works. In routine practice, the use of background infusions as well as PCA does not improve analgesia and increases side effects such as sedation and ventilatory depression. Background infusion may be indicated in patients who have been taking high dose opioids before PCA was used, for example those with long-term cancer pain.

Local, regional and spinal analgesia

Local blocks

Some simple nerve blocks and injections can provide excellent symptomatic relief with minimal discomfort and risk for the patient with acute pain. Most simple blocks can be performed with local anaesthetic, quite basic equipment and attention to asepsis in a clean environment. Minimal aftercare is usually needed. Patients may experience transient motor weakness for the duration of the local anaesthetic, and they must be warned to protect the limb during this time.

- Dental nerve blocks are the most commonly used local analgesic technique for restorative dental care and they can also be used to treat acute dental pain.

- Suprascapular nerve block can be very useful in patients with shoulder pain either alone or as an adjunct to intra-articular shoulder injection for acute shoulder pain.

- Simple upper limb blocks such as to the ulnar, radial or median nerve can be used to treat nerve entrapments or analgesia for procedures.

- Ilioinguinal and iliohypogastric nerves may be blocked to treat nerve entrapments, postoperatively or for pain in surgical scars.

- Femoral nerve block may be useful in patients with pain in the hip or to reduce muscle spasm in patients with femoral fractures. This approach can be useful for incident pain or as a temporary measure whilst waiting for other treatment.

- Intra-articular injections can be used for a variety of joint pains such as shoulder, hip or knee; these are simple to perform. Intra-articular injection during arthroscopy may also be useful for postoperative analgesia. Opioids can be injected into inflamed joints but the evidence base for this practice is small.

- Lower limb blocks such as to the common peroneal and tibial nerves may be used to treat nerve entrapments or provide analgesia for procedures.

Regional blocks

A variety of regional nerve blocks that allow interruption of individual nerve plexuses or ganglia can be used for managing pain. These are usually more technically demanding than the peripheral nerve blocks and simple injections. They often have more serious potential complications. Regional nerve blocks must be undertaken only with adequate facilities including skilled assistance, sterility, monitoring, equipment, appropriate imaging, resuscitation and aftercare. Infusion techniques using catheters may be needed for long-term use, for example after surgery. In patients with breakthrough or incident pain, catheter techniques may be used to give boluses of drugs before stimuli that provoke pain.

Brachial plexus blocks can be used for arm pain. The dose of local anaesthetic required is large and the potential for adverse effects exists.

Intercostal blockade can be used to treat unilateral, well-localized chest wall pain within a few dermatomes. There is a risk of pneumothorax, especially in very slim patients, in obese patients where the ribs cannot be felt or in those who have had chest surgery that may make the pleura adherent. Multiple blocks should be avoided. Intercostal blocks result in higher plasma local anaesthetic concentrations than any other technique because of rapid absorption from the muscle and subpleural space. It is therefore important that the toxic dose is not exceeded.

Intrapleural or paravertebral analgesia may be preferable if several dermatomes are affected. Although the effect of local anaesthetic alone is often brief, the technique may be used to provide analgesia in the acute situation, such as rib fractures.

Lumbar plexus can be blocked where it passes via the psoas compartment and this provides analgesia for the hip and leg. The technique is simple and safe. A single injection of local anaesthetic can be used – or an infusion of local anaesthetic can provide a more prolonged effect.

Lumbar sympathetic block can be used to treat ischaemic vascular leg pain.

Spinal analgesia

Spinal analgesia is useful in acute pain. Single injections of local anaesthetic and steroid can be used to manage a variety of conditions. A thorough working knowledge of spinal anatomy is essential for all practitioners involved in caring for patients receiving spinal drugs. It is important that staff understand the distinction between:

- Intrathecal (subarachnoid) drug delivery into cerebrospinal fluid (CSF)
- Epidural drug administration into the more superficial epidural space.

Drug doses and the risks of some complications differ between these two routes. Complications of spinal analgesia include: drug-related side effects (e.g. motor blockade, emesis, itching), permanent neurological damage (0.05–0.005%), transient neuropathy (0.013–0.023%), epidural haematoma (1 in 100 000), epidural abscess (0.015–0.05%), meningitis, ventilatory depression (<2%), hypotension (<5%) and failed analgesia.

Intrathecal techniques Intrathecal injection can be performed from the cervical to the lumbar region. The dura terminates at a variable level, usually at S2 in adults, but in some cases reaching S4/5 (the dura extends more caudally in children). It is therefore possible accidentally to enter the subarachnoid space during caudal epidural injection. It is preferable to perform any injection below L2 where the spinal cord normally terminates in an adult; this reduces the risk of direct spinal cord damage. Local anaesthetics and opioids can be given intrathecally after surgery to provide analgesia for the first 24 hours after surgery.

Epidural techniques The epidural space is largely a potential space, bounded superiorly where the periosteal and spinal layers of the dura fuse at the foramen magnum. Therefore, drugs injected epidurally do not usually pass intracranially. The epidural space continues inferiorly to the sacrococcygeal membrane where it is entered during caudal epidural block. Epidural injection or cannulation can be performed at any level from cervical to sacral; different levels require slightly different techniques and have different risks and benefits. The analgesia produced by an epidural infusion depends on the level chosen for injection or catheterization and the volume of solution infused.

Single epidural injections are simple and relatively safe. Epidural steroids are probably effective in single dose in the short term for lumbosacral, radicular pain. Epidural catheters can be used to infuse drugs in patients with a variety of acute pains (e.g. labour pain, acute trauma or postsurgical pain). Epidural infusions provide better analgesia than parenteral opioids and may improve surgical outcomes; for example in high risk patients the use of thoracic epidurals reduces pulmonary complications and myocardial infarctions. Drugs must be infused from dedicated pumps that are fit for the purpose. These must have a large capacity and the ability to give low volume infusions with precision. Each unit must standardize the pumps used so that staff training and maintenance of equipment are as simple as possible. Education about the equipment used is essential. Spinal drug delivery will fail if staff education is neglected. Where the appropriate resources are not available, then spinal techniques must not be used.

Drugs used in local, regional and spinal analgesia

Local anaesthetics *Indications* These can be used to provide analgesia for acute pain during local and regional blocks. Spinal analgesia can be provided by an infusion of low dose local anaesthetic. When comparing spinal local anaesthetics a minimum local anaesthetic concentration (MLAC) can be found where 50% of patients achieve satisfactory analgesia. Studies have not shown a consistent difference in efficacy when long-acting local anaesthetics are used; the usual concentrations of these for postoperative pain or labour are 0.1–0.2%. When infusions are used then systemic toxicity is rare; but there is still the potential for problems if accidental large boluses or intravenous administration occurs. Epidural PCA has been used in obstetric and postoperative analgesia with some success. In labour, epidural PCA reduces local anaesthetic dose, motor block and the number of anaesthetic interventions needed (e.g. bolus doses).

Pharmacology All local anaesthetics have a similar chemical structure with a lipophilic aromatic ring linked to a hydrophilic moiety by a carbon chain. They prevent nerve conduction by blocking sodium channels in axonal membranes. Nerve transmission also depends upon the structure of the nerves. Individual fibres vary in their degree of myelinization, speed of conduction and susceptibility to blockade. The block produced by application of a local anaesthetic is influenced by the relative position of the fibres within a nerve bundle, the outermost fibres being blocked first. Usually the susceptibility to blockade is predictable. Sympathetic nerves are blocked more easily than pain, temperature and touch fibres that are more susceptible than pressure, proprioception and motor nerve fibres. It is possible to produce analgesia without motor block, but if analgesia is present then sympathetic block will usually occur.

The clinical effects of local anaesthetics depend upon their physicochemical properties. The individual volume and con-centration of the drug is unimportant; for example 60 mg of lidocaine gives the same result whether given as 3 ml of 2% or 6 ml of 1%. However, an increase in the volume administered may sometimes affect the block by extending the spread of local anaesthetic.

Potency increases with increased lipid solubility; for example bupivacaine is lipid soluble and is more potent than the less soluble lidocaine. Their speed of onset is related to the degree of ionization of the drug at body pH, diffusibility of the drug across membranes and the concentration gradient devel-oped between the site of injection and the site of action. Local anaesthetics are weak bases that are poorly soluble in water. The base diffuses to the site of action; however, the cation is the active agent. As the tissue pH falls, local anaesthetics become more ionized and less diffusible. Therefore, they cannot get to the site of action in acid conditions (e.g. infection). Local anaesthetics are more readily absorbed from inflamed areas, and injection into vascular sites increases the risk of a toxic reaction.

Their duration of action increases with increased protein binding and is influenced by the intrinsic vasoactive effect of the drug. The duration of action of local anaesthetics also depends upon the rate of removal from the site of action by bulk flow during injection, and diffusion that is influenced by local blood flow. Local anaesthetics with large chemical groups (e.g. bupivacaine) resist hydrolysis, and they are therefore longer acting. Renal excretion of unchanged local anaesthetics is minimal.

The site of injection alters the speed of onset and duration of the block; for example subcutaneous infiltration anaesthesia begins rapidly and is short lived, but plexus anaesthesia often starts slowly and may last for many hours.

Lidocaine is the drug of choice for short procedures, but is not useful for long-term infusions as it produces less effective analgesia and more motor block than the longer-acting agents such as bupivacaine, levo-bupivacaine and ropivacaine. There are no consistent differences in quality of analgesia and motor blockade with the long-acting local anaesthetics.

Epinephrine can be added to local anaesthetics to increase the speed of onset and duration of action and reduce bleeding. Concentrations of more than 5 µg/ml (1 : 200 000) are not necessary and can lead to toxicity (the maximum safe dose of epinephrine for a healthy adult is 500 µg). A high concentration of epinephrine (1 : 80 000) is commonly used in dental anaesthesia. The use of epinephrine increases the duration of action of short- and intermediate-acting local anaesthetics by inducing local vasoconstriction, but differences are less apparent with long-acting agents. Epinephrine decreases plasma levels and toxicity when added to lidocaine, but the effect on bupivacaine absorption is less. It reduces local bleeding, if sufficient time (10–15 minutes) is allowed to elapse between injection and incision. Epinephrine must not be used near end arteries such as digits, nose, penis or pinna, nor for intravenous regional anaesthesia. It should be used with caution in patients with thyrotoxicosis, hypertension, ischaemic heart disease, peripheral vascular disease or phaeochromocytoma. It can safely be given to patients taking monoamine oxidase inhibitors.

Side effects It is important to calculate the toxic dose of local anaesthetic allowed in each patient and to stay well within the dose limit. Systemic toxicity of local anaesthetics is a continuum that depends on blood, myocardial and brain drug concentrations. Systemic toxicity commonly occurs owing to inadvertent intravascular injection or administration of too high a dose. The main toxic effects are central nervous and cardiovascular. The cardiovascular system is four to seven times more resistant to these effects, so seizures will usually occur before cardiovascular collapse. The myocardial toxicity of bupivacaine is long lasting and difficult to reverse. It is more toxic to the central nervous and cardiovascular systems than the other two long-acting drugs that are its structurally related isomers. Large doses of bupivacaine should be avoided. Outcomes are more favourable and resuscitation from overdose more likely with ropivacaine.

Opioids *Indications* Opioids can be administered spinally for many acute pain indications.

Pharmacology They produce analgesia via pre- and postsynaptic receptors in the spinal cord and brain. Lipid solubility is important when choosing a spinal opioid; water-soluble drugs have a greater relative potency than the more lipid soluble agents. For example fentanyl acts more quickly, but is of shorter duration than the hydrophilic drugs such as morphine.

Adverse effects All spinal opioids can cause respiratory depression, sedation, confusion, emesis, constipation, retention of urine and itching. Morphine remains in cerebrospinal fluid for longer, rather than penetrating the cord and nerve roots, so it may spread cephalad and be more likely to cause ventilatory depression. Therefore patients who have received spinal opioids require careful monitoring for 24–48 hours afterwards; this is especially important in opioid-naive patients.

Other spinal drugs Multimodal spinal analgesia allows the use of lower doses of individual drugs and limits side effects (e.g. local anaesthetic and opioid together). Other drugs such as clonidine, baclofen, neostigmine and ketamine have been used spinally for acute pain management. The side effects of these drugs may differ from those of local anaesthetics and opioids. The evidence base for routine use of many of these drugs is poor.

Non-pharmacological analgesia

Transcutaneous electrical nerve stimulation (TENS)

Indications and use of tens Many acute pain problems (e.g. musculoskeletal pain, dysmenorrhoea and labour) have been treated with TENS. The aim is to produce an area of paraesthesia that must completely cover the area of pain. In many pain conditions, standard electrode positions can be suggested on a dermatomal basis. Trying different combinations of electrode positions and settings for each patient is often required. The evidence from trials investigating the role of TENS in acute and postoperative pain management remains inconclusive. The number of well-conducted randomized controlled trials is small. There are some unique obstacles to rigorous TENS research and studies have often used flawed methodology. Blinding is difficult in clinical trials; patients and staff are quick to notice the presence or absence of paraesthesia in the appropriate area. If studies are not blinded the treatment effect may be exaggerated by up to 17%. Inadequate randomization can exaggerate the treatment effect by up to 40%. Different forms of TENS may not be comparable. Timing, electrode placements and duration of stimulation are important variables. There is a placebo response to TENS. The evidence for the clinical effectiveness of TENS in acute pain is not clear; it may help in primary dysmenorrhoea. It is relatively cheap and free from harmful side effects, compared with many pain interventions; this has led to its increasing use without rigorous scientific evaluation. Future research may reveal it to be an effective treatment for some conditions, possibly mild–moderate postoperative pain, but ineffective for others, as has been shown for labour and severe postoperative pain.

Mode of action The effects of TENS are complex. Electrical stimulation excites $A\beta$ afferent nerve fibres connected to tactile receptors, these enter the spinal cord and ascend in the dorsal columns; $A\beta$ afferents also give collaterals in the spinal cord. The collaterals synapse with short interneurons, ending near C-fibre terminals that synapse in the substantia gelatinosa. The interneurons release gamma amino butyric acid (GABA). Presynaptic blockade of the C afferents occurs via GABA thereby preventing them from exciting the substantia gelatinosa cells and so 'closing the gate'.

Tens equipment This consists of a battery-operated stimulator with connecting leads and skin electrodes that are applied to produce paraesthesia covering an area of pain. Machines need to be compact, lightweight, hard wearing, portable, fitted with two channels and able to stimulate with four electrodes. Electrodes are self-adhesive, disposable conductive pads with a life span of 10–14 days. Stimulators should have adjustable amplitude and frequency controls that are capable of generating continuous and pulsed patterns.

Different modes of tens These include continuous (40–150 Hz, 10–30 mA), which causes non-painful paraesthesia in the stimulated area, pulsed (bursts of 100 Hz at 1–2 Hz, 10–30 mA), which produces non-painful paraesthesia felt as bursts in the stimulated area, and acupuncture-like TENS (bursts of 100 Hz at 1–2 Hz, 15–50 mA), with non-painful muscle twitch in the myotome stimulated. The different forms of TENS do not produce the same physiological effects. The duration and timing of TENS stimulation are other variables. Intermittent stimulation for short intervals (e.g. 30 minutes) may be more effective than prolonged or continuous stimulation; the development of tolerance may reduce effectiveness. It takes 20–30 minutes for analgesia to develop and plateau. It takes about 45 minutes for pain thresholds to return to baseline values following cessation of stimulation.

Complications of tens These include skin irritation, minor electrical burns and allergy to the electrode material. Equipment failure is uncommon. Problems more often arise from failure to understand instructions about how to use TENS.

Psychological interventions

(See Ch. 18.)

Self-assessment questions

Answer 'True' or 'False' to the following statements:

15.1 Acute pain causes:

    a. Catabolism
    b. Hypoglycaemia
    c. Increased gluconeogenesis
    d. Reduced blood coagulability
    e. Sodium and water loss

15.2 Postoperative pain causes:

    a. Hypoxaemia
    b. Atelectasis

   c. Ileus
   d. Hypotension
   e. Myocardial ischaemia

15.3 Number needed to treat (NNT) is:

   a. Used to compare analgesics
   b. High for effective therapies
   c. Decreased when analgesics are combined, e.g. para-cetamol and codeine
   d. Variable between patients
   e. Usually similar to the number needed to harm (NNH)

15.4 Paracetamol:

   a. Affects peripheral cyclo-oxygenase synthesis
   b. Is a useful anti-inflammatory drug
   c. Causes peptic ulceration
   d. Does not affect platelet function
   e. Is as well absorbed after rectal administration as after oral dosing

15.5 Effects of NSAIDs are:

   a. Gastrointestinal bleeding
   b. Bronchodilatation
   c. Reduced renal blood flow in shocked patients
   d. Hypotension
   e. Hypercoagulability

15.6 Morphine:

   a. Is absorbed better than hydromorphone after oral dosing
   b. Has analgesic metabolites
   c. Is best given as a controlled release formulation for acute pain
   d. Is contraindicated in renal colic
   e. Is a full agonist at opioid receptors

15.7 Intravenous patient-controlled analgesia (PCA) systems:

   a. Allow patients to regulate their own pain relief
   b. Increase risk of ventilatory depression on general wards
   c. Have an optimum bolus dose in adults of 10 mg for morphine
   d. Provide better analgesia than intravenous infusion
   e. Do not reduce opioid consumption

15.8 Complications of spinal analgesia include:

    a.   Motor blockade

    b.   Itching

    c.   Jaundice

    d.   Permanent neurological damage

    e.   Hypertension

15.9 Which of the following is likely to reduce postoperative pain to the greatest extent following an abdominal procedure?

    a.   Prescription of a standard analgesic to be given as required

    b.   The use of patient-controlled analgesia administered intravenously

    c.   Postoperative counselling and preparation by relaxation

    d.   Acupuncture postoperatively

    e.   Hypnosis postoperatively

Management of chronic non-cancer pain

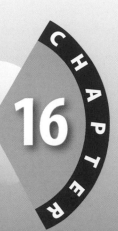

CHAPTER 16

Chapter objectives

After studying this chapter you should be able to:

1 Understand the nature of chronic non-cancer pain and recognize different examples of chronic pain conditions.

2 Know about the adverse physical, psychological and social effects of chronic pain on the patient and their carers.

3 Know about systemic analgesics for chronic pain management and the use of different routes of drug administration.

4 Know about local, regional and spinal analgesia for chronic pain management.

5 Know about neuromodulation for chronic pain.

6 Understand the role of non-pharmacological physical interventions for chronic pain.

7 Understand the role of psychological therapies for chronic pain.

The nature of chronic pain

Unrelieved persistent pain is a major problem for patients and a massive socioeconomic burden for the health service and community. There are many causes of chronic pain (Table 16.1). These cause interference with daily activities, especially in younger patients. This may lead to depression, psychological problems, prolonged disability and problem drug use. It leads

Table 16.1 Examples of chronic non-cancer pain conditions

Type of condition	Examples
Musculoskeletal	Cervical spondylosis
	Degenerative low back pain
	Osteoarthritis
	Rheumatoid arthritis
	Myofascial pain syndromes
Post-traumatic	Brachial plexus injury
	Vertebral crush fractures
Postsurgical	After breast surgery
	After hernia repair
	After thoracotomy
	After amputation
Central nervous	Multiple sclerosis
	Spinal cord damage
	Poststroke
	Syringomyelia
Peripheral nervous	Peripheral neuropathy
	Complex regional pain syndrome
Facial pain	Trigeminal neuralgia
	Temporomandibular joint pain
Headaches	Tension headache
	Migraine
	Cluster headaches
Post-infection	Postherpetic neuralgia
Vascular	Peripheral vascular disease
Visceral pain	Pancreatitis
	Mesenteric ischaemia
	Refractory angina
Urogenital pain	Postvasectomy
	Endometriosis

to significant use of medical services and increased costs to the taxpayer. Chronic pain is associated with older age, perhaps female gender, low socioeconomic status, poor education, poor general health, increased psychological distress and unemployment. It is also a problem in children and adolescents perhaps affecting up to 25%. Patients with chronic pain often present with complex physical and psychosocial problems that require multidisciplinary management. Patients who are referred to pain clinics most commonly present with musculoskeletal pain (e.g. back pain). Neuropathic pain is less common, but often more difficult to manage. Headache and visceral pains are also commonly seen.

Efficient and effective pain management requires close links between medical specialties (e.g. surgery, medicine, rheumatology, gastroenterology, neurology, elderly medicine, rehabilitation medicine, occupational health, oncology, palliative medicine, psychiatry, addiction medicine, paediatrics and primary care). Good pain management needs interdisciplinary cooperation between healthcare professionals (e.g. doctors, specialist nurses, clinical psychologists, physiotherapists, pharmacists and occupational therapists).

Effects of chronic pain on patients, their carers and society

Chronic pain has a profound effect on the quality of life of patients and their families:

- Studies suggest that 11–30% of people have significant chronic pain problems and that these problems persist for many years.
- The young working population are commonly affected, and a large study showed that the average age of those with chronic pain was 49 years.
- A third of patients described their pain as so bad that they could not tolerate any more pain.
- About 50% of people with chronic pain feel tired all the time, helpless, or older than they really are, and do not remember what it feels like not to be in pain.
- One in five say the pain is sometimes so bad they want to die.
- One-third reports that their pain affects employment; one in four reports losing a job owing to pain.
- About a quarter have depression because of their pain.

The economic burden of musculoskeletal problems is also high:

- It accounts for 1–2.5% of the gross national product of many Western countries.

- Back pain is one of the top 10 most expensive problems.

- A 1998 UK survey showed that, during a 12 month period, 40% of adults suffered from an acute attack of back pain lasting more than 1 day, and nearly 40% of these people presented to their general practice.

- About five million adults consult a doctor about back pain every year.

- About a third of those aged 16–24 years old reported 1–6 days of back pain during a 1 year period.

- In 1998, in the UK, the direct healthcare cost of back pain was £1632 million, and the cost of informal care and lost production was £10 668 million.

- In Europe, persistent pain leads to about 500 million lost working days per year and costs in the region of 34 billion euros.

Therefore, persistent pain is a big problem, and finding effective treatments has important clinical, social and economic implications. Specialist pain management services provide clinically effective care at a low cost when compared with many other secondary care services. However, as persistent pain is so common, it is clear that most pain management happens in primary care. Therefore, community-based services need education and information about pain management strategies.

Analgesics for chronic non-cancer pain

Multimodal therapy (see Ch. 4) is more effective than monotherapy, so it is important to emphasize that pharmacological therapies should be seen as only a part of an integrated management plan to improve physical and social function. All healthcare professionals involved in managing persistent pain should address behaviours and coping styles that increase disability and dependence. Drugs must only be used to facilitate rehabilitation that should involve setting clear goals, with plans for steady progress towards them. There are many systematic reviews on the use of analgesic drugs and techniques (e.g. the Oxford Bandolier Pain website and the Cochrane site).

It is essential to balance the benefits and burdens of drug treatment carefully because chronic pain may require long-term medication. Effective relief of pain is obtained with oral drugs; therefore it is important to use the most effective and safest oral analgesics available. The use of injectable analgesics in chronic pain must be discouraged, as this approach often creates more problems than it solves. There are some situations where transdermal drug delivery offers advantages such as convenience, and less requirement to think about medication several times each day.

Simple analgesics and weak opioids

Paracetamol remains the first line simple analgesic. It should be taken regularly up to the maximum adult dose of 4 g/day; patients must be warned about the risks of exceeding this dose. Paracetamol 1 g has an NNT of nearly 5; combining it with codeine 60 mg improves analgesia. Weak opioids perform badly when given alone; combining them with simple analgesics improves their efficacy. However, long-term use of codeine causes significant constipation that needs to be managed actively. The use of weak opioids such as dihydrocodeine can escalate in patients with persistent pain; problem drug use and diversion of drugs for illicit use can occur. Prescribers need to be aware of this and they should monitor patients' behaviour when these drugs are used long term. Demands for increasing doses and a daily use outside the prescribed dose range may be causes for concern.

NSAIDs and COX-2 inhibitors

Oral NSAIDs do very well in single dose postoperative comparisons. However, this does not consider adverse effects, and these are particularly important in chronic use in the elderly. The adverse effects of NSAIDs are appreciable and well known. About 1.9% of NSAID users in one area in the UK were admitted to hospital urgently each year with upper gastrointestinal problems; the duration of NSAID use was not important. Emergency admissions in the UK that were attributable to NSAID-related adverse events were about 12 000 per year with about 2500 deaths, the risk increasing with increasing age. There may also be an increased risk with certain drugs such as piroxicam and ketorolac. The NSAIDs cause renal impairment and can cause congestive cardiac failure; age is the major co-risk factor. Topical NSAIDs are effective and do not have gut side effects; they have an NNT of about 3 in chronic conditions.

COX-2 inhibitors may offer partial solutions. Their analgesic potency is equivalent to the best analgesics presently available. In osteoarthritis and rheumatoid arthritis, their analgesic efficacy is similar to NSAIDs. Therefore, the deciding issue on choice of treatment is adverse effects. COX-2 inhibitors have a good safety profile for gastrointestinal complications compared with NSAIDs. Data on endoscopic ulcers suggest that COX-2 inhibitors have a similar incidence to placebo. The balance of evidence is that serious bleeding is also no more likely with COX-2 inhibitors than with placebo. However, they still cause renal problems and their long-term effect on cardiovascular risks such as stroke is not clear and is a cause for concern.

Strong opioids

Indications Only 10–15 years ago, opioids were thought to be useless as long-term therapy for chronic pain. It was suggested that analgesia would be lost to tolerance and dependence would be common. It was formerly believed that all neuropathic pains were totally morphine insensitive. More recent clinical research has shown that, although centrally mediated neuropathic pain at cerebral and brain stem level may be refractory, more peripheral neuropathic pains may be partially responsive to opioids. Therefore, there is a continuum of opioid responsiveness in various chronic pain states at clinically tolerable doses. In the early 1980s, these views were challenged, mainly by uncontrolled retrospective reports of efficacy of opioids long term for non-cancer pain and neuropathic pain with little dose escalation and low dependence. Patients tolerate long-term opioid treatment only if it either produces good analgesia or improves function. Indications for opioids are about pain severity and its impact on life, not about diagnosis. The focus should be on efficacy, adverse effects and safety in long-term use, rather than the legal and abuse issues that seem to dominate thinking.

Current opinion is that, in some patients with persistent non-cancer pain, strong opioids can provide analgesia and perhaps improve quality of life without leading to escalating doses or problem drug use. There are very few adequate randomized controlled trials of prolonged opioid therapy on which to base practice. Therefore, prescribers must exercise judgement when considering this treatment. Patients with persistent pain can often have poorly defined conditions, difficult behavioural problems and unsupportive social situations. The long-term consequences of opioids in this setting are understood poorly. Pain management must be the primary goal when opioids are used, and not anxiolysis or sedation. Improvements in sleep, physical, psychological and social function may occur secondary to opioid analgesia.

Pharmacology (see Ch. 15) Morphine is usually the drug of first choice and should be given as the oral modified release preparation. The transdermal route is a possible option. Skin patches are easy to use, with few complications and a long duration of action. Fentanyl and buprenorphine are suitable for transdermal administration as they have a low molecular weight combined with high potency and lipid solubility. Patches are applied every 72 hours. A small number of patients may need patches changing every 48 hours for pharmacokinetic reasons; such patients may need specialist pain management during dose finding. Initial dose titration is slow, as transdermal drugs take a long time to achieve steady-state plasma concentration (at least three half-lives). However, once this is attained, patches often prevent 'clock watching' and many breakthrough problems. It may also allow patients to get on with their lives and forget about medication. Patches can be very useful in patients who cannot take oral medications, for example those with gastrointestinal problems.

All opioids were seen as the same when given in equipotent doses; this is not true. If one opioid does not work, then it is important to try a different one; this is called 'opioid switching'. It is common to need to reduce the dose when switching between opioids. Action at other receptors may also be important; for example methadone acts at NMDA and tramadol at 5HT receptors.

Adverse effects Opioid side effects are inevitable; these must be managed promptly (see also Ch. 15). Disadvantages specific to skin patches include difficulty with rapid dose variation in response to circumstances; this route should not be used in those with pain that is changing quickly or for incident or breakthrough pain. If side effects occur then they are often not quickly reversed, as a drug depot remains under the skin for many hours after the patch has been taken off. Some patients cannot tolerate patches because of skin irritation. Rotating the patch site and using local steroids can often manage this, but sometimes patients have to abandon patches.

Concerns about patients' behaviour, tolerance, dependence, and addiction are a factor in the reluctance to use opioids in non-cancer pain. These definitions are out of context in the prescribed use of opioids for pain.

- Tolerance is uncommon when opioids are used for persistent pain; the majority of patients stabilize on a long-term dose after a period of dose titration that may take several months.

- Physical dependence is common in patients using a stable opioid dose; it is not clinically important if opioid withdrawal is medically supervised.

- Psychological dependence is compulsion to use the drug; it is probably rare when patients are appropriately prescribed a stable dose of opioid for pain management.

- Addiction means the compulsive use of opioids to the detriment of the user's physical and/or psychological health and/or social function. It is not possible to use screening tools such as questionnaires to predict the likelihood of addiction for individual patients. The use of opioids prescribed for pain probably only rarely results in addiction. Many studies suggest that the risk is small.

- Pseudoaddiction describes behaviours such as drug hoarding, attempts to obtain extra supplies and requests for early prescription or increased dose. These are not always manifestations of true addiction; they cease when pain is managed properly.

If problem drug use occurs in the context of treating persistent pain, then it is important to recognize it quickly and act appropriately. Concern that a patient's behaviour may indicate addiction should trigger immediate referral to/consultation with a specialized drug addiction unit.

Several countries worldwide have reported problems when opioid prescribing has become too ubiquitous in these circumstances. It is partly for this reason that many countries have produced written recommendations about the use of opioids for persistent non-cancer pain, and common themes emerge (Box 16.1). Recommendations for prescribing and patient information are available in the UK from the British Pain Society website. Medicine is about relative risks and benefits, and it remains to be seen how opioids will fit in with other treatments.

Adjuvant analgesics

Antidepressants Antidepressants are effective in reducing neuropathic pain by diverse pharmacological actions, for example inhibition of presynaptic norepinephrine and 5-HT reuptake, postsynaptic activity at a variety of sites, NMDA receptor blockade, and sodium and calcium channel blockade.

- Older less specific drugs such as amitriptyline are more effective than the newer drugs that target fewer receptor sites such as fluoxetine. The NNT for at least 50% of pain relief for tricyclic antidepressants compared with placebo is

Box 16.1

Recommendations for strong opioid prescribing in persistent non-cancer pain

- Appropriate assessment of pain.
- Close working relationships between primary and secondary care.
- Opioids considered only after established therapies.
- Doctor to make initial decision to use strong opioids.
- Extended prescribing possible by other healthcare professionals.
- Acute pain teams not to initiate long-term opioids without support.
- Individual treatment plans.
- Patients made aware of limitations/side effects of opioids, and their responsibilities.
- Psychological comorbidity, social chaos or history of alcohol/ problem drug use does not absolutely preclude use of opioids.
- Written information for patients about opioids.
- Modified release or transdermal opioids preferable.
- Immediate release formulations avoided.
- Injectable opioids rarely appropriate.
- Patients eventually to obtain medication from single source usually in community.
- Primary outcome pain relief.
- Secondary aims of demonstrable improvements in physical, psychological and social function.
- Regular assessment in primary and/or secondary care.
- Documented evaluation of: pain relief, physical, psychological and social function, sleep, side effects, signs of problem drug use.
- All healthcare professionals alert to risk of drug diversion.
- Local protocols developed.

2–3 for most pain conditions. Many of the trials demonstrated analgesic benefit without significant changes in mood. The starting dose should be low (e.g. 10 mg amitriptyline at night) and titration should be supervised and slow. Side effects include sedation, blurred vision, dry mouth, increased appetite and constipation. At higher doses, cardiac arrhythmias, postural hypotension, urinary and sexual problems can occur. The NNH for minor adverse effects is 2–3 based. For major effects, the NNH is about 17.

- Tricyclic antidepressants are more effective for pain than selective serotonin reuptake inhibitors that have an NNT of 6–7. Venlafaxine has been shown to be effective for postsurgical neuropathic pain, for example after breast surgery.

Anticonvulsants

There is good evidence that anticonvulsants are useful in managing diabetic neuropathy and PHN. There is preliminary evidence that anticonvulsants are useful in a number of other pain conditions, but this is based on single trials.

- Carbamazepine has been used for trigeminal neuralgia for many years. It has an NNT of 2–3 in a dose of 300–2400 mg per day. About 10% of patients cannot tolerate treatment owing to side effects such as dizziness, ataxia and sedation. It may be useful in other neuropathic pain conditions. Patients' haematological and liver function tests are required.

- Sodium valproate has been used for migraine and has an NNT of 3.5. It is also used for neuropathic pain, but there is little efficacy evidence. It has significant side effects, for example nausea, dizziness, sedation and ataxia with an NNH for stopping the drug due to side effects of 9.

- Gabapentin is an anticonvulsant that has antihyperalgesic and antiallodynia properties, but does not have significant actions as an antinociceptive agent. Its mechanisms of action appear to be complex synergy between increased GABA synthesis, non-NMDA receptor antagonism and binding to the voltage-dependent calcium channels. Clinically, several large randomized controlled trials have demonstrated its effectiveness in the treatment of a variety of neuropathic pain syndromes. Patients with neuropathic pain gain a mean reduction in pain score of 2.05 points on an 11 point numerical rating scale compared with 0.94 points if they had taken placebo. Around 30% of patients achieve more than 50% pain relief. A similar number will also experience minor adverse events; the most common of which are somnolence and dizziness. Three of the four major trials in neuropathic pain demonstrate no differences between study withdrawals in those taking placebo compared with those taking gabapentin.

- Pregabalin is a newer anticonvulsant that is similar to gabapentin but has the advantage of twice daily dosing.

- Lamotrigine is an anticonvulsant that blocks sodium channels and inhibits glutamate release. It is effective for trigeminal neuralgia (NNT 2) and poststroke pain, but its use for other neuropathic pains remains unproven. It has some troublesome side effects and it is often poorly tolerated.

Comparisons of antidepressants and anticonvulsants

Information from meta-analyses and systematic reviews allows comparisons of effectiveness of drugs in various neuropathic pain conditions. In postherpetic neuralgia, the NNT for gabapentin was 3.2 that compared with 2.3 for tricyclic antidepressants and 2.5 for oxycodone. In diabetic neuropathy, the NNTs are: gabapentin 3.8, tricyclic antidepressants 3.0 and carbamazepine 2.3. In diabetic neuropathy studies, the NNH for minor events is 2.5 for gabapentin, 3.7 for carbamazepine and 2.8 for tricyclic antidepressants. The NNH for major events (drug-related withdrawal from study) is 20–40; this is broadly similar for tricyclic antidepressants and anticonvulsants (excluding gabapentin). The relatively high risk for minor adverse effects of anticonvulsants should be considered when prescribing long term.

Membrane stabilizers

Intravenous lidocaine has been shown to be effective for neuropathic pain. Mexilitine has been given orally to try to produce a more sustained effect; there is no evidence to support its efficacy and side effects are a problem.

Ketamine

The NMDA antagonist ketamine has been used orally to manage a variety of difficult pain problems. It is metabolized to norketamine, which is probably the active analgesic. There can be problems with patients obtaining this drug in the community. It has psychomimetic side effects and long-term use requires careful ongoing assessment.

Cannabinoids

Pharmacology The major active component of Cannabis sativa is Δ-9-THC. Marijuana is prepared from the dried flowering tops, stalks, seeds and leaves (Δ-9-THC 0.5–5.0%), hashish is dried resin/compressed flowers (Δ-9THC 2–20%) and hashish oil is extracted by organic solvents (15–50% Δ-9-THC). It is highly lipid soluble and can be absorbed easily from the lungs (5–24% bioavailable) and gut (6% bioavailable). The plasma elimination half-life of Δ-9-THC is about 56 hours in occasional users and 28 hours in chronic users. Cannabis is metabolized in the liver to more than 20 metabolites, some of which are active and have long half-lives. Metabolites can be excreted by the liver and gut (35–65%), and to a small extent the kidneys (15–30%). Complete elimination of a single dose may take 30 days.

Effects on pain Cannabinoids act at specific G-protein-coupled receptor sites in both neuronal (CB1) and peripheral tissues (CB2). Cannabinoids and opioids probably act on similar areas of the CNS, but their action is mediated via different receptor systems. The potent analgesic effect of cannabinoids in animals and the presence of CB1 receptors in pain-processing areas of the CNS suggest that endogenous cannabinoids may contribute to the control of pain transmission. There is also evidence that they can also modify pain transmission by a peripheral action on CB1 and CB2 receptors, thus there may be a possibility for peripherally administered cannabinoids as analgesics. The discovery of cannabinoid receptors led to the synthesis of non-selective ligands (e.g. levonantradol and nabilone).

- Nabilone has been used in chronic pain. It has a shorter half-life than Δ-9-THC. Withdrawal reactions have been seen after prolonged use. At high dose it may have a more euphoria effect than Δ-9-THC.

- There is a long history of therapeutic use of cannabis in many cultures, including for analgesia. There is little clinical trial evidence relating to the analgesic effects of cannabinoids, but there is very strong and recent basic science literature in support of efficacy.

- Clinical trials show that the efficacy of currently available cannabinoids is modest; they have an unfavourable therapeutic index and bioavailability problems; the transmucosal route may offer some solutions to this. Most of the trials are based on either the main psychoactive ingredient of cannabis (Δ^9 tetrahydrocannabinol) or closely related compounds.

- A systematic review of trials published up to 1999 identified nine clinical trials of cannabinoids of sufficient quality for analysis. Five of these trials used cancer pain as a model, whilst two used chronic non-malignant pain and two acute pain. The overall analgesic effect of cannabinoids was approximately equivalent to codeine 50–120 mg.

- Adverse effects were common in all studies.

- There are also concerns about the long-term risk of developing mental illness in regular cannabis users that are relevant for the patients taking cannabinoids long term.

- The limited evidence published to date does not support a role for cannabis in the control of pain.

Topical preparations

- In patients with allodynia the application of a film dressing to the area (e.g. Tegaderm) may be helpful.
- Topical NSAIDs may be helpful for patients with chronic musculoskeletal pain. They have few side effects.
- Lidocaine patches can be helpful for patients with postherpetic neuralgia and arthritis. Lidoderm 5% contains lidocaine 700 mg in a 20 × 15 cm patch; it can be cut to size and worn for 12 hours each day. However, in the elderly they can be difficult to use, 30% get skin reactions, and this preparation is not readily available in many countries.
- Capsaicin is an alkaloid derived from chillies that acts to deplete substance P in local nerve sensory terminals. Topically applied capsaicin (0.025 and 0.075%) is useful in alleviating the pain associated with diabetic neuropathy, osteoarthritis, postherpetic neuralgia, stump pain and scar pain. The numbers-needed-to-treat for some improvement are 3–6. However, the inconvenience of regular topical application and the local burning that it produces make patient compliance with treatment difficult.

Local, regional, spinal and interventional techniques for chronic pain management

Patients with chronic pain have complex biopsychosocial problems that cannot be addressed with unimodal therapy; pain services should provide the whole range of treatment options. Nerve blocks should form part of a strategy aimed at pain management, functional restoration and rehabilitation. There is no point in using physical techniques alone to manage pain that has significant non-physical elements. Nerve blocking is used to manage chronic pain, but it must be seen in the context of a multidisciplinary approach to pain management.

A careful assessment at the outset will avoid subjecting a patient to an invasive procedure with little chance of benefit. Decision making is dependent on good communication both within a team and between teams when a nerve block or neuromodulation technique is being considered. Interventions may need to be performed urgently, but are rarely needed as an emergency. It is important that patients are given time to think about the options and to ask questions; written information can be very helpful.

The techniques offered depend on the skills and resources of the local pain management service. Most nerve blocks and neuromodulation techniques are performed under local anaesthetic, but patient comfort and cooperation are of great importance, so sedation or general anaesthesia may be needed. The operator may sometimes give simple sedation, allowing verbal contact with the patient to be maintained throughout. This is only possible where there are trained staff members available to monitor the patient during the procedure. When the procedure is to take place under general anaesthesia or heavy sedation, the anaesthetic must be given by a separate anaesthetist; there is no situation that justifies a single operator–anaesthetist.

The availability of appropriate pain management facilities is essential. Where a specialist pain service is available, there is usually access to anaesthesia, theatres, imaging, day-case facilities and beds. Where there is no such service, then invasive techniques are not an option. Undertaking complex interventions in suboptimal conditions is not worth the risk. Referral to another specialist centre for more complex interventions (e.g. epiduroscopy) may sometimes be appropriate. However, referrals for techniques that need ongoing management, such as spinal drug delivery, may not be appropriate if local follow-up and aftercare is not available.

Nerve blocks may be a single injection or may involve the placement of a catheter with an infusion of drugs from a pump. There are several situations where nerve blocks may form part of treatment (Table 16.2).

- Simple nerve blocks can be performed in a clinic setting, for example myofascial trigger spot and intra-articular injections.

- Complex techniques are usually performed in an operating theatre and may require image intensification, for example paravertebral blocks and lumbar sympathectomy. The success rate of some more complex blocks may be improved by the use of a peripheral nerve stimulator and insulated needles. Electrical stimulation is then used to locate the needle tip close to nerves and nerve plexuses, for example brachial plexus block.

Table 16.2 Examples of nerve blocks for chronic non-cancer pain conditions

Condition	Nerve block
Musculoskeletal	Trigger point injections
	Intra-articular injections
	Paravertebral blocks
	Epidurals
	Dorsal root blocks
	Facet joint injections
Post-traumatic	Brachial plexus block
	Lumbar plexus block
	Guanethidine blocks
Postsurgical	Scar injection
Facial pain	Trigeminal radiofrequency lesions
	Gasserian ganglion block
	Stellate ganglion block
Headaches	Botulinum toxin trigger point injections
Vascular	Lumbar sympathectomy

- Spinal blocks can be useful, for example single epidural or caudal injections of local anaesthetic and steroid can be used to treat a variety of conditions. Single epidural injections are simple and relatively safe. Epidural steroids are probably effective in the short term for lumbar, non-cancer, radicular pain. There is little evidence for their use in malignant nerve root pain; however, many case reports and series suggest good results.

Drugs used for local, regional and spinal blocks

- Single injections usually use local anaesthetic, e.g. long-acting agents (levo-bupivacaine and ropivacaine).
- Hydrocortisone is a weak anti-inflammatory agent that is absorbed quickly and has an effect that often lasts only a few days.
- The synthetic steroids such as triamcinolone hexacetonide, triamcinolone acetonide or methylprednisolone acetate are about five times more potent and less soluble; their effect can last weeks or months. Systemic absorption after injection may be sufficient to reduce inflammation in areas that have not been injected. High or repeated doses may

suppress the hypothalamic–pituitary–adrenal axis. Injections should not be repeated more often than every 8–12 weeks. There is controversy about the use of depot steroids epidurally, but there is no animal or clinical evidence that they are neurotoxic in the doses administered.

- Opioids may be used peripherally and there is some evidence that opioids are effective analgesics when they are injected into joints.

- Botulinum toxin may be used to treat painful muscle trigger spots and spasticity.

- Chemical neurolysis with phenol, ethyl alcohol and glycerol are only appropriate for conditions such as vascular pain or trigeminal neuralgia. Neurolytics should not be used in other non-cancer pains.

Radiofrequency lesions

Radiofrequency lesions are performed using fine probes that are placed on the target area. A stimulating current is passed down the probe to check its position by inducing appropriate sensory effects and ensuring that motor nerves are not stimulated. The patient needs to be awake and cooperative for this to be successful. Local anaesthetic is injected down the probe before lesioning is performed. Pulsed radiofrequency lesioning can be used when the probe does not reach a high temperature, but it is thought that the radiofrequency current itself has an analgesic effect. Reinnervation is almost inevitable after any radiofrequency technique but usually takes some months; the procedure can be repeated.

This technique is not appropriate for peripheral nerves, as it can lead to increased pain after reinnervation and deafferentation pain. It is used to treat musculoskeletal pain such as that coming from spinal facet joints and sacroiliac joints. It can also ablate the lumbar sympathetic chain in peripheral vascular pain.

Complex interventions

Interventions that are more complex are usually performed in specialist centres. Many do not yet have a solid evidence base to support their routine use. Many of these techniques are best done as part of ongoing clinical trials to establish their place in treatment.

- Epiduroscopy involves passage of a fibreoptic instrument into the caudal canal. It is advanced cephalad to treat epidural nerve root adhesions.

- Vertebral fractures from the midthoracic to lumbar region can be treated by vertebroplasty; this requires injection of bone cement via a needle into the vertebral body.

- Intradiscal thermal nucleolysis involves passing a heating coil under fluoroscopy into a vertebral disc to lesion the disc.

Spinal cord stimulation (SCS)

The spinal gate concept gave rise to SCS, where electrodes are placed in the epidural space and electrically simulated using an implanted pulse generator. SCS is a treatment with a supportive evidence base that has been used for the treatment of pain since 1967. The relationship of SCS to gating mechanisms remains unclear.

Its aim is to reduce the unpleasant sensory experience of pain and the consequent modification of experience and behaviour. When it is used to treat patients with chronic pain it must be delivered with a full understanding of the impact that pain has upon the patient, the extent that pain interferes with their life and how it impacts on their psychological well-being. SCS should be delivered within services that can offer comprehensive assessments and a range of additional physical and psychological treatments. The clinical management team needs to be involved in selecting patients for SCS. A variety of factors must be considered:

- Pathology (Box 16.2)

- Area of pain – a large area may increase the number of electrodes implanted and the complexity of the system programming; some areas are difficult to target selectively such as low back, perineum and genitalia

- Pain type – SCS is most successful in neuropathic pain

- Life expectancy – the patient must have an adequate life expectancy SCS to be beneficial

- Previous and current therapy

- Planned therapy or investigations – e.g. MRI may be difficult with a spinal electrode

- Psychological issues – patients should be assessed by a clinical psychologist before considering SCS.

An electrode is placed in the epidural space under local anaesthetic, and then a pulse generator is placed in the abdomen to provide the stimulating current. During electrode placement, the patient tells the operator whether the correct

Box 16.2

Indications for SCS

Good indications for SCS (likely to respond)

- Brachial plexopathy: traumatic, postirradiation
- Complex regional pain syndrome
- Neuropathic pain in limb (e.g. FBSS)
- Peripheral vascular disease
- Refractory angina

Intermediate indications for SCS (may respond)

- Amputation pain
- Axial pain following spinal surgery
- Intercostal neuralgia
- Spinal cord damage
- Perineal, anorectal pain
- Peripheral neuropathic pain syndromes

Poor indications for SCS (rarely respond)

- Central pain of non-spinal cord origin
- Spinal cord injury with complete loss of posterior column function

Unresponsive to SCS

- Complete spinal cord transection
- Non-ischaemic nociceptive pain
- Nerve root avulsion

electrode position has been achieved, so that paraesthesiae are produced over the whole area of pain. The electrode position and configuration chosen should cover the widest dermatomal area, so that if the pain spreads the stimulation pattern may be altered. A second electrode can be introduced to increase stimulation.

Patients have local pain after the procedure. The most serious complication of SCS is infection. If this occurs in any part of the system, the complete unit must be removed and antibiotics given. The most common later problems are: electrode migration, dislodgement, lead fracture and current leakage. When used with the correct indications, and by experienced practitioners, SCS can be beneficial and cost effective for patients with complex pain.

Intrathecal drug delivery (ITDD)

Infusing analgesics or antispasmodics directly to spinal receptors offers excellent analgesia or muscle relaxation, or both, in carefully selected patients with non-cancer and cancer pain, and some neurological conditions. A variety of drugs can be placed in the intrathecal space to provide analgesia (e.g. opioids). Muscle relaxants can also be used to reduce spasticity (e.g. Baclofen). ITDD can reduce the burden of systemic drug side effects in some patients. ITDD should be used selectively; it is appropriate for only a small number of patients. It should be considered when simpler, safer and more economical methods have been tried and failed. Before ITDD, patients should usually undergo spinal imaging to exclude surgical pathology at the level of the intended ITDD catheter placement. Careful assessment of physical, psychological and social factors are important when considering ITDD. Detailed explanation of the benefits and burdens of ITDD is required before patients can take the decision to embark upon this treatment.

A multidisciplinary pain management team is the most appropriate context for delivery of ITDD. The team must have established relationships with the other teams involved in the patient's care. The team will usually comprise several professionals, for example a consultant in pain medicine, one or more consultants from other relevant specialties (e.g. palliative medicine, neurology, rehabilitation medicine, neurosurgery, spinal surgery, cardiology, vascular surgery, radiology), a clinical psychologist, pharmacists, physiotherapists specializing in pain management and clinical nurse specialists in pain management and palliative care. It is important to develop regional and national recommendations about the context in which ITDD is delivered and the techniques used. Standardization of drug choices, doses, preparation and presentation may be helpful. It is particularly important to have robust systems for aseptic preparation.

All intrathecal drugs produce side effects that should be monitored and managed. Sedation, confusion or hypotension may necessitate dose changes or drug switching. Emesis is usually temporary and should be managed using standard therapy; if it persists then drug switching may be needed. Itch from opioids may be treated (e.g. with ondansetron). Long-term intrathecal opioid use has endocrine and immune effects;

the significance of these is not clear. Altered sexual function may occur, which may respond to hormonal treatment. Sensory or motor blockade with local anaesthetics should be adequately managed; this may require reduction in local anaesthetic dose, which is not always possible without loss of analgesia.

Non-pharmacological physical interventions

Various physical interventions are used to manage chronic pain. Most have the advantage of avoiding drug side effects and promoting patients' self efficacy. Physiotherapists, occupational therapists and specialist nurses have important roles in delivering many of these therapies. Other healthcare practitioners may also be involved, for example osteopaths, chiropractors and acupuncturists. Some strategies rely on mobilizations and exercise. An important part of this is teaching patients with pain about regular, paced exercise and reducing maladaptive behaviours such as fear–avoidance. Other therapies may involve stimulation of the nervous system, for example transcutaneous electrical nerve stimulation (TENS) or acupuncture.

The mechanism underlying the action of TENS on the spinal cord is shown in Figure 16.1.

TENS

Meta-analyses of randomized controlled trials of TENS produced several conclusions. None of the TENS trials were blinded, although this is much more difficult than blinding in drug studies. Outcome measures should be about pain intensity or pain relief. Indirect measures such as the need to use other analgesic interventions or a reduction of analgesic consumption are less useful. The dose of TENS used must be adequate. There is a lack of evidence for the effectiveness of TENS at recommended treatment schedules. At lower treatment schedules in which TENS is used only intermittently or for short periods, there is no evidence that TENS provides effective pain relief. More prolonged use of TENS in chronic pain might be justified, although this remains to be proven.

Acupuncture

Acupuncture began to appear in the English medical literature about 150 years ago. Interest declined over the early part of the last century and has re-emerged in the past 40 years. In

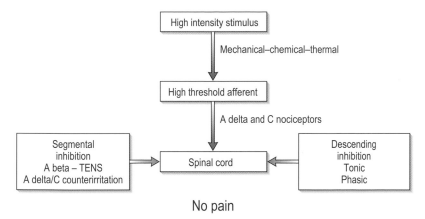

Fig 16.1 Blocking of high intensity stimuli (A delta and C nociceptor neurons) by suppression of dorsal horn cells using TENS stimulation of A-beta neurons. Reproduced from Textbook of Pain 3 edn, Wall PD & Melzack R (Eds), Churchill Livingstone, 1994.

1995, a survey of 8745 people found that 1 in 4 used complementary medicine (12% of these used acupuncture). This compares with a similar survey in 1986 that showed 1 in 12 people were using complementary therapy. Acupuncture is popular again; two studies of adverse events during acupuncture surveyed about 66 000 acupuncture treatments in the UK during a relatively short time scale. The use of acupuncture is widespread in the USA where in 1998 it was estimated that more than a million Americans have acupuncture each year.

The usual approach is based on a combination of segmental point selection, trigger point therapy, and the use of some traditional Chinese points. There are various types of stimulation that can be used for acupuncture, such as acupressure, manual needling, electrical stimulation or laser stimulation. Various frequencies and intensities of stimulation have different effects on the release of neurotransmitters. Sometimes acupuncture is used in specific areas, as in auricular treatment. Some patients are more sensitive to acupuncture than others, and can be described as strong reactors. Trigger point therapy is used for a wide variety of musculoskeletal and visceral disorders. A segmental approach to treatment relevant to the affected dermatomes, myotomes and sclerotomes can be used. Strong traditional analgesic points such as Large Intestine 4 on the dorsum of the hand and Liver 3 on the foot are often used.

Complementary therapies need to be evaluated carefully. The test of time is insufficient evidence upon which to base therapies. Rigorous assessment of efficacy is as important for acupuncture as for any other treatment. Acupuncture should be integrated into routine care only if it is proved to be effective after proper evaluation. Over the past 10 years, there have been several large systematic reviews of acupuncture published. A Cochrane field devoted to complementary medicine has been established. There are four well-supported indications for acupuncture using the available evidence: dental pain, low back pain, migraine and emesis. There are many indications where a large number of randomized controlled trials have been published, but systematic reviews are inconclusive (e.g. addiction, headache and neck pain). The evidence for acupuncture efficacy for treatment of smoking and obesity is conclusively negative.

Psychological therapies for chronic pain
(See Ch. 18.)

Self-assessment questions

Answer 'True' or 'False' to the following statements:

16.1 Back pain:

    a. Is one of the top 10 most expensive healthcare problems

    b. Occurs acutely for more than 1 day in 20% of adults annually in the UK

    c. In young adults usually requires radiological investigations

    d. Is rare in patients less than 25 years of age

    e. Leads to 500 million lost working days per year in Europe

16.2 Paracetamol:

    a. When taken in a dose of 1 g by an adult as an NNT of nearly 5

    b. Analgesia is improved when it is combined with a weak opioid

    c. Has more side effects than NSAIDs

    d. Should be avoided in patients with a history of alcohol abuse

    e. Should be avoided in children under 12 years

16.3 Strong opioids:

    a. Should only be prescribed long term for patients with cancer pain

   b. Commonly cause physical dependence
   c. Commonly lead to addictive behaviours when pre-
       scribed for chronic pain
   d. Lead to emesis that usually resolves after a few
       weeks of treatment
   e. Lead to constipation that usually resolves after a few
       weeks of treatment

16.4   Antidepressants:
   a. Are effective in managing neuropathic pain
   b. Reduce pain by altering mood
   c. In the tricyclic group have NNTs above 6
   d. Cannot be used long term in pain management
   e. Can be combined with simple analgesics

16.5   Cannabinoids:
   a. Are clinically useful analgesics
   b. Reduce painful muscle spasm in a dose-dependent
       manner
   c. Are poorly absorbed after oral dosing
   d. Have a short elimination half-life
   e. Have active metabolites

Management of cancer pain

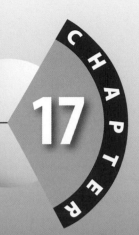

C H A P T E R

17

Chapter objectives

After studying this chapter you should be able to:

1 Understand the incidence and nature of pain in cancer and gain a working knowledge of basic assessment and management for cancer pain.

2 Understand the place of appropriate investigations and disease modification.

3 Understand that psychosocial and spiritual supports are components of total care.

4 Appreciate the need for physical treatments in some patients.

5 Understand the basic principles of pharmacotherapy for cancer pain.

6 Appreciate the need for more complex interventions for those with difficult cancer pain, and what these interventions involve for the patient, e.g. nerve blocks, neuromodulation, radiological interventions and surgery.

7 Understand that certain groups may have particular needs, e.g. children, those with cognitive impairment and problem drug users.

Pain in cancer – the nature of the problem

The incidence of cancer in adults continues to rise worldwide and despite significant advances in treatment, many cancers remain incurable. Pain in cancer is one of the most feared symptoms; it will affect most patients at some stage during their illness. The prevalence of pain in cancer varies with the nature of the cancer, the stage of the disease (Fig. 17.1) and the methods used for assessment:

- Approximately 30–40% of patients with cancer on active therapy report pain.
- This rises to 70–90% of patients with advanced disease.
- More than 50% of patients in hospitals and hospices have pain.
- Approximately one-third have a single pain, one-third have two pains and one-third have three or more pains.

There are many causes for pain in patients with cancer (Box 17.1); 85% of pain is due to the cancer itself, and 15% is caused by general debility, a concurrent disorder or treatment:

- Breakthrough pain is that which breaks through good pain control from background analgesia. It can usually be successfully managed by increasing the dose of background drug treatment.
- Incident pain occurs predictably given a particular stimulus, for example movement-related pain of bone metastases. Incident pains can be acute, severe and disabling and are often short lived; they do not respond well to oral analgesics.

Fig 17.1 Advanced cancer of the breast.

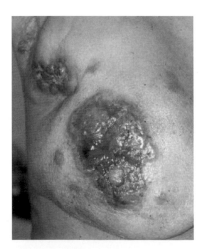

> **Box 17.1**
>
> ## Causes of pain in cancer
>
> **Pain from the cancer**
>
> - Visceral, e.g. liver capsule pain, bowel obstruction
> - Somatic, e.g. bone metastases
> - Headache, e.g. meningeal disease
> - Neuropathic, e.g. plexus invasion
>
> **Cancer treatments**
>
> - Chemotherapy, e.g. mucositis, peripheral neuropathies
> - Postlumbar puncture headache
> - Radiotherapy, e.g. radionecrosis
> - Surgery, e.g. wounds/drains, phantom limb pain
> - Drugs, e.g. NSAID-induced gut ulceration
> - Investigations, e.g. stenting or biopsy
>
> **General debility**
>
> - Infections
> - Reduced mobility/weight loss, e.g. joint pain and stiffness, pressure sores or deep venous thrombosis
>
> **Non-cancer pain**
>
> - Ischaemia, e.g. ischaemic limb pain
> - Musculoskeletal, e.g. osteoporotic fractures
> - Neuropathic, e.g. AIDS related or diabetic neuropathy
> - Headache, e.g. tension headache

- Procedural pain is a particular type of incident pain that predictably occurs during a procedure, such as dressing changes.
- Increasing the dose of background drugs causes sedation when pain is not present, and nerve blocks can be particularly useful in the management of these difficult pains.

Cancer pain management principles

Pain management depends on a logical approach, assessing and treating each cause of pain. Comprehensive pain assessment is essential. There are many cultural differences in the presentation of painful disease, reaction to life-threatening illness and response to therapies that should be taken into account during assessment. The concept of 'total pain' encompasses physical aspects of pain with its psychological, social and spiritual dimensions; patients' and carers' distress should also be addressed. Optimal pain management depends on assessment of:

- Precise details about the pain(s)
- Comorbid and premorbid medical problems
- Physical function
- Psychosocial and spiritual factors.

Accurate characterization of the pain or pains is important, including location, severity, quality, temporal factors and aggravating/relieving factors. Some patients also find it helpful to keep a pain diary. Grading the intensity of pain using a simple numerical rating scale (0–5) or as none, mild, moderate or severe at rest, in relation to activity and to therapeutic interventions can help. Pain scales are available in many languages and may be downloaded and printed with English translations, available from the British Pain Society (www.britishpainsociety. org). A history of medication use is needed, including assessing the effects and side effects of analgesics at different doses and by different routes.

An increase in pain intensity following a stable period necessitates prompt evaluation of the underlying aetiology. Rapidly escalating pain is an emergency that requires prompt assessment and intervention. Common emergencies in patients with cancer who present with pain are pain due to spinal cord compression and pathological fractures; these conditions need prompt evaluation and treatment.

Factors other than pain form an important part of assessment; these include:

- Physical symptoms (e.g. fatigue, nausea, anorexia, and constipation)
- Coexistent psychological symptoms
- Psychiatric disorders (e.g. anxiety and depression)
- Functional status
- Family dynamics
- Spirituality
- Social support systems
- Medical support systems
- Financial resources.

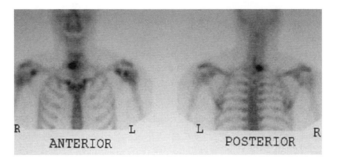

Fig 17.2 Bone scintiscan showing secondary tumour deposits in the skeleton of a patient with carcinoma of the breast.

Evaluation of cancer pain requires a full physical examination, a review of laboratory and radiographic tests, and further investigations such as ultrasound, radioisotope (Fig. 17.1), CT and MRI, with biopsy if appropriate. Cancer pain is often associated with structural pathology, and this may not always be obvious with available imaging techniques. Definition of the extent of disease and the nature of the underlying aetiology of pain is essential to pain assessment. However, diagnostic tests should be ordered only if the information contributes to the plan of care and it is consistent with the patient and family's goals of care. Otherwise, treatment may be empirical, especially at the end of life. The patient's goal is often for cancer therapy, but it is important to recognize when anticancer treatments are no longer appropriate.

Management must involve:

- Treating the cause of the pain where possible, for example appropriate use of antibiotics for infection, fixation for fractures and spinal stabilization
- Modifying the disease process if possible, for example palliative radiotherapy/chemotherapy, bisphosphonates for hypercalcaemia, and surgery for bowel obstruction
- Dealing with factors exacerbating the pain; for example in patients with dyspepsia, NSAIDs should be withdrawn or replaced with COX-2 inhibitors.

Oral or parenteral administration of primary and secondary analgesic drugs is the mainstay of pain management for most patients with cancer. Physical methods of treatment such as physiotherapy, peripheral neural stimulation (TENS or acupuncture) may be of value. Specialized management techniques such as simple or complex nerve blocks, neuromodulation or neurosurgery may be needed for selected patients with pain that is difficult to control. There is a spiritual element to many patients' pain, and this needs exploring; for example worsening symptoms may suggest the progression of disease and impending death to patients and carers. Attention to a patient's physical environment is vital for the holistic management of pain. Simple measures such as use of appropriate mattresses, orthotics and mobility or bathing aids can enhance comfort. Mood disorders are common in patients with cancer. Depression and anxiety may worsen a patient's pain experience; this should be diagnosed and treated.

Psychological approaches to cancer pain

Pain that has significant non-physical elements will often not respond to physical treatments used in isolation. A careful assessment at the outset will avoid subjecting a patient to an invasive procedure with little chance of benefit. Patients with cancer pain often have a variety of psychological and psychosocial concerns that require a comprehensive assessment; depression and anxiety are common. Care givers also suffer distress. Spiritual problems are important in some patients and families. Clinical psychologists, psychiatrists and trained counsellors may be helpful. A variety of cognitive interventions, such as relaxation, guided imagery and cognitive behavioural therapy, may be used to improve pain control or coping with pain.

Most (90%) of a patient's cancer care occurs at home. Attention to the patient's and carer's social environment is also important; there should be a seamless transition from hospital to home care with palliative care units (hospital palliative care teams and community-based hospices) acting as a link between the two. Good communication within and between teams is essential.

Physical therapies for cancer pain

Physiotherapists and occupational therapists are useful team members in cancer pain assessment and management. Interventions include:

- Prevention of secondary myofascial or joint complications in patients with weakened limbs
- Local heat or cold
- Massage

- Orthotics
- Stimulatory approaches (e.g. counterirritation)
- TENS
- Acupuncture.

Many of these are used empirically for some patients with cancer pain. A strong evidence base does not support these at present, but they have the advantage of being non-invasive. Rehabilitation can be an important part of pain management in cancer, when these professionals can play a key role.

Analgesic drugs for cancer pain

Analgesic pharmacotherapy is the mainstay of cancer pain management. Optimal oral drug regimens manage more than 75% of patients with cancer pain if basic principles are followed:

- Drugs should be given orally whenever possible.
- Drugs should be given regularly rather than on demand.
- Regular analgesics and coanalgesics should be prescribed using the WHO analgesic ladder (Fig. 17.3). This method of drug selection involves starting with simple analgesics and moving up the ladder if pain does not improve.

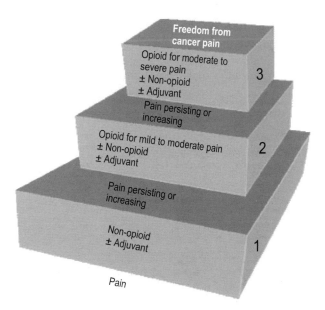

Fig 17.3 World Health Organization analgesic ladder. Adapted from Cancer pain relief: with a guide to opioid availability, 2edn. Geneva: World Health Organization, 1996.

- Other coanalgesics, for example antidepressants, anticonvulsants, NSAIDs with a proton pump inhibitor or cyclooxygenase-2 inhibitors should be used in parallel if necessary.

Non-opioid analgesics including regular oral paracetamol are used first (step one). If this is not effective then weak opioids combined with the simple analgesics are needed for moderate pain, for example codeine, oxycodone (combined with a non-opioid analgesic in a single preparation), dihydrocodeine and tramadol (step two). If weak opioids do not help, there is no point in switching to another weak opioid, and the next step up the ladder is needed. Patients with severe cancer pain require strong opioids, for example morphine, hydromorphone, oxycodone (used alone), methadone, fentanyl, buprenorphine and diamorphine (step three).

Lack of opioid availability in some countries and poor education of doctors and nurses about the rational use of strong opioids is still a serious impediment to effective pain management. There is evidence that some healthcare professionals still hesitate before prescribing strong opioids for patients with severe cancer pain. This is often due to lack of knowledge about pharmacotherapy or groundless fears about opioid side effects and addiction. Such opioiphobia is very detrimental to optimal analgesia and results in much unnecessary suffering worldwide. There is never a need to withhold strong opioids from those with severe pain from cancer.

Strong opioids

Morphine This is the strong opioid of first choice in most situations. It is a μ agonist that acts in the brain and spinal cord. Morphine is well absorbed from the upper gut, but its extensive metabolism by the liver leads to a reduced oral bioavailabilty. Morphine is available in several different preparations:

- Immediate release tablets or liquid provide rapid analgesia of brief duration (about 4 hours). This formulation is useful for dose finding and acute exacerbations of pain.
- Modified release preparations (tablets, capsules or suspension) are useful; they allow twice-daily dosing. They should not be used for titration and are not helpful for acute pain.

Strong opioid dose should be reviewed regularly and titrated to achieve optimum pain control:

- Morphine should initially be given orally every 4 hours, and the response monitored closely to allow rapid titration to achieve analgesia.

- There is no maximum dose, the amount required is determined by pain relief and limited only by side effect; however most adults need less than 200 mg morphine daily.

- Doses should be increased until adequate analgesia occurs or intolerable and unmanageable side effects supervene; for example it is usually necessary to increase the dose of morphine by 30–50% each time.

- The absolute dose is not important as long as a favourable balance between analgesia and side effects is maintained.

- Initially it is often easier to titrate the dose of strong opioids by using immediate release formulations every 4 hours.

- Once pain control has been achieved, then modified release formulations that can be given every 12 hours are more convenient.

- It is also important that patients have drugs prescribed for breakthrough pain and that these are immediate release formulations.

- Patients with stable disease seldom need to increase their opioid dose; if this occurs it suggests recurrent or progressive disease.

- Morphine has an active metabolite, morphine-6-glucuronide that can accumulate in patients with renal failure, so that dose reduction or another opioid may be needed.

Other strong opioids Various alternatives to morphine may be useful when it produces limiting side effects such as nausea, confusion or drowsiness. Opioid switching may be used to achieve better pain control and fewer side effects.

- Fentanyl is a strong μ agonist and buprenorphine is a partial agonist; both are available as a transdermal patch with duration of effect of 3 days. These may be helpful in stable pain situations, but cannot be used for titration or acute breakthrough pain. They are useful for patients who cannot swallow or absorb oral drugs. They produce less constipation than morphine. Fentanyl is also formulated as an oral transmucosal lozenge that can be used for rapid pain control in breakthrough pain. The dose needed cannot be predicted from knowledge of the prior opioid dose; it needs to be carefully titrated.

- Oxycodone and hydromorphone are alternative strong opioids that are available as immediate and modified release preparations.

- Methadone is a longer-acting strong agonist with some slightly different properties; it has to be given 8 hourly or less and it can accumulate.

- Pethidine and propoxyphene should not be used for cancer pain management; their side effects outweigh the benefits.

- When drugs are given subcutaneously using a syringe driver, then diamorphine is very useful because it is so lipid soluble and can be given in small volumes.

Opioid side effects   Common opioid side effects must be managed promptly to optimize therapy:

- Antiemetics are often needed initially (haloperidol and cyclizine may be useful), but patients usually become tolerant to opioid-related emesis within 3–4 days of regular treatment.

- Constipation usually persists; appropriate aperients and bowel care should manage it.

- Drowsiness is common but often gets better after the first few days of therapy.

- Ventilatory depression is not usually a problem. It may occur if patients are treated with high dose opioids, and then given a simultaneous pain-relieving procedure, e.g. a nerve block. In this situation, the dose of opioids should usually be reduced.

- All patients taking regular opioids will develop withdrawal symptoms if the drugs are stopped abruptly. Opioids should be slowly reduced before discontinuation of therapy and antagonist drugs should be avoided.

- Problem drug use is a psychological and behavioural disorder characterized by loss of control over drug use, compulsive drug use, and continued drug use despite harm; this is rare during opioid treatment for cancer pain.

Adjuvant analgesics

Many other analgesics are used to treat cancer pain and symptoms, including:

- Antidepressants (e.g. amitriptyline, nortriptyline, venlafaxine)

- Anticonvulsants (e.g. gabapentin, pregabalin, sodium valproate, carbamazepine)

- Local anaesthetics (applied topically)

- Miscellaneous drugs (e.g. ketamine, baclofen, clonidine)
- Cannabinoids – however there is poor evidence that their efficacy is good and the side effect burden is high; they should be used in parallel with the analgesic ladder
- Corticosteroids – to treat nerve swelling, liver capsule pain and headache from raised intracranial pressure; a high dose is needed in the latter case (dexamethasone is used because it is much more potent than prednisolone; it should usually be given as a short course of treatment)
- Anticholinergic drugs (e.g. scopolamine)
- Antisecretory drugs (e.g. octreotide) – for colicky pain from malignant bowel obstruction
- Haloperidol and midazolam – these are important in the management of terminal restlessness and agitation; at the end of life opioids, haloperidol and midazolam are commonly given subcutaneously using small syringe drivers for patients who are too ill to take oral drugs.

Nerve blocks and neuromodulation

About 10–15% of patients with cancer-related pain can be helped by nerve blocks. Nerve blocks should not be regarded as a treatment given in isolation but must form part of an overall strategy for analgesia. Nerve blocks are often left as a last resort, by which time the patient may be too ill to tolerate the technique or to come to a hospital for the more complex procedures. Careful selection of patients and timing of interventions are vital. Early discussion with colleagues in pain management services is essential. It is important that staff looking after patients with cancer can recognize pains that can be managed by nerve blocks and understand what each procedure entails so that appropriate and timely referrals can be made. Decisions about aftercare need to occur before any intervention is considered. Some contraindications to nerve blocks include:

- Physical frailty
- Local or systemic sepsis (especially indwelling system)
- Neutropenia/thrombocytopenia
- Concomitant medication (anticoagulants) and impending spinal cord compression or raised intracranial pressure, where a spinal block is being considered
- Lack of capacity to make an informed choice.

There are basic principles in using these for the management of pain from cancer (Box 17.2):

Box 17.2

Principles of nerve blocking in patients with cancer

- Early referral for consideration of interventions.
- Appropriate expertise and facilities available.
- Clear communication within and between teams.
- Total pain carefully assessed.
- Appropriate laboratory tests, radiology and neurophysiology performed.
- Nerve blocks must not cause functional defects.
- Neurodestructive procedures must be selective of sensory or autonomic nerves and leave motor paths and sphincters intact.
- Careful explanation to ensure the full understanding and consent of the patient.
- Patients and carers given adequate time to ask questions.
- Aftercare organized with staff who understand the nature of the procedure, what it can and cannot achieve, how to look after the patient and the likely effects and side effects.

- It is best to start with simple peripheral nerve blocks and progress to more complex regional blocks later.
- The simplest methods possible should be used to manage pain, and all available alternatives to an invasive technique should be considered.
- Simple nerve blocks may be easy to organize and readily accepted by the patient; these may be done at home or in the hospice. Examples include trigger point or intra-articular injections of local anaesthetic and steroids.
- If pain is widespread or disease is progressing rapidly, it is unlikely that simple blocks will produce long-term benefit. It is then sometimes better to perform a more definitive procedure rather than put the patient through multiple different blocks.
- When more complex blocks or infusion techniques are considered, patients require careful evaluation and multiprofessional team members need to be involved in decision making. Optimal oral analgesia may be more acceptable if the alternative is a complex nerve block requiring hospital admission and extensive aftercare.
- The patient must be carefully informed of the anticipated benefits and likelihood of complications of all techniques.

Every intervention must be considered in terms of its possible benefits, what is needed of the patient, carers and staff, inconvenience, risks and recuperative time.

- Referrals for techniques that need ongoing management, such as spinal drug delivery, may not be appropriate if local follow-up and aftercare are not available (see Ch. 16).

Spinal drug delivery

Drugs can be given spinally either as single injections epidurally or intrathecally, as a single dose of intrathecal neurolytic or by external or internal spinal infusions. Single doses of epidural local anaesthetic and steroid may help with nerve root pain and pain from vertebral collapse. Intrathecal neurolytic delivery may help perineal pain or tenesmus; however, it carries risks to bladder and bowel function, so careful patient selection is essential. More complex pain problems are best served by spinal infusions. Pain in the head may be managed by intracerebroventricular drug delivery with the help of a neurosurgeon.

Surgical and interventional radiological approaches to cancer pain

Sometime surgery for those with cancer can provide analgesia, for example repair of bowel obstruction, stabilization of pathological fractures in long bones and spine, and vertebrectomy for metastatic disease. Stenting is another technique that can provide pain control in visceral obstruction. Some neurosurgical procedures may be useful for cancer pain, for example rhizotomy and cordotomy. In those with head and neck cancer, intraventricular drug delivery might be considered. Adequate performance of the actual procedure is a small part of the total management of the patient's pain. Explanation and consent are needed when considering surgery in this situation. Patients and carers need time to assess the benefits and burdens of surgery in this situation.

Radiotherapy

Palliation of cancer pain by radiotherapy is often very effective, for example with painful bony metastases and fungating lesions. It is important that the patient understands that radiotherapy usually does not work immediately, and that pain may get worse initially from tissue swelling. Sometimes a nerve block can be used to deal with the pain whilst waiting for radiation to take effect. Side effects from radiation must be managed appropriately and quickly (e.g. mucocytis, skin problems and diarrhoea). It is important that radiotherapy is planned to disrupt the patient's life minimally, for example keeping the number of fractions of radiation treatment as low as possible.

Special populations with cancer pain

- The needs of children with cancer pain are different to adults. Age-appropriate assessments, appropriate staff training and attention to environment are all important. There is little provision at present for specialist paediatric pain management and palliative care. Drug doses must be adjusted for age and weight. Non-drug therapies may be particularly applicable. Interventional analgesic techniques may be useful, but will usually involve sedation or anaesthesia.

- Those with learning difficulties with cancer pain may need assessment and communication can be difficult.

- The needs of the elderly with cancer pain may include different psychosocial concerns. Cognitive impairment in the elderly and other comorbidities may alter drug handling in this group. Polypharmacy is a particular problem, and changes in drug selection and dosing needed because of age-related variation in pharmacokinetics and pharmacodynamics.

- Problem drug users who have cancer pain can be particularly hard to manage. There is a requirement for closer monitoring of drug use and an increased likelihood of under treatment. Drug withdrawal may occur and needs active management. Referral to specialists in addiction medicine may be helpful.

Self-assessment questions

Answer 'True' or 'False' to the following statements:

17.1 Pain:

    a. Occurs in 50% of patients with advanced cancer

    b. Occurs in more than 50% of those in hospices

    c. Occurs in a single site in 70% of patients with cancer

    d. In patients with cancer is always caused by the malignancy

    e. That occurs only on movement is called incident pain

17.2 Analgesic drugs used for cancer pain management:

    a. Provide relief in less than 50% cases

    b. Should be used when necessary rather than given by the clock

    c. Should usually be combined with sedatives

    d. Should be given orally where possible

    e. Should be withheld until the patient has a short life expectancy

17.3 Morphine:

    a. Is the strong opioid of choice in cancer pain

    b. Is a full μ agonist

    c. Is poorly absorbed after oral administration

    d. Has active metabolites

    e. Causes constipation that improves within a few days of starting treatment

17.4 Nerve blocks:

    a. Can be useful in 10–15% of patients with a cancer pain

    b. Should be considered only when all other options have been tried

    c. Are contraindicated by irreversible coagulopathy

    d. Can usually be performed at the bedside

    e. Have few side effects

17.5 Radiotherapy:

    a. Has no place in pain control

    b. Always works quickly

    c. May be used to treat painful bone metastases

    d. Has minimal morbidity

    e. May be used to treat painful fungating lesions

Psychological techniques in pain management

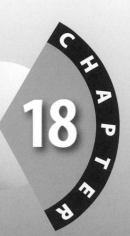

18

Chapter objectives

After studying this chapter you should be able to:

1 Understand the psychological approach to the management of pain through individual techniques.

2 Describe psychological techniques of pain management.

3 Appreciate the reasons for the different uses of psychological techniques of pain management.

Psychological methods used for pain reduction

This chapter is divided into several sections, each describing a method of psychological treatment (Box 18.1) and should be read in conjunction with Chapter 5. The decision to use any of these techniques almost always follows a period of medical assessment. Referrals are made then to a clinical psychologist or other therapist working in a family practice, or as part of a multidisciplinary, hospital-based team, (acute pain team, palliative care team or pain management team practising multimodal therapy, which is a combination of physical and psychological methods of management). Occasionally the referral is to a clinical psychologist or counsellor working alone. This is often less favourable because a partnership between a doctor and a therapist dealing with a patient who usually regards the problem as physical adds credibility to the process for the patient. The partnership facilitates good communications between the professionals.

The work of the therapist may involve a one-to-one relationship with a pain patient, working with patient groups or some combination of both methods, and at all times requires well-developed communication skills (Box 18.2). A fuller explanation of the work of other pain management team members was given in Chapters 15 to 17.

Relaxation

Relaxation is a technique that reduces tension, anxiety and pain. Once taught it can be practised without further need for

---

Box 18.1

Psychologically based pain management

- Relaxation
- Hypnosis
- Biofeedback
- Cognitive/behavioural therapy
- Counselling
- Interpretative therapy – individual
- Group/family therapy

(The use of psychotropic drugs for psychological and/or analgesic purposes may be an aspect of management.)

> **Box 18.2**
>
> ## The nature and value of communication skills
>
> - Good clinician/patient communication is central to effective practice.
> - Poor communication increases the risk of inaccurate diagnosis, patient dissatisfaction and failure to cooperate with treatment.
> - There are several important factors influencing the effectiveness of clinician/patient communications and they include:
>   - the physical setting/the interchange
>   - verbal communication skills
>   - non-verbal communications
>   - the psychosocial context of the interaction, including the effect of a clinician's personal characteristics upon the patient and vice versa.
> - Effective clinical communication requires the ability to use the relevant skills flexibly in response to the needs of different patients.

a trainer. This gives the patient a feeling of control over tension and pain and that is a major benefit of the therapy.

There are several techniques for inducing relaxation:

1   *Diaphragmatic breathing*. The patient should be seated comfortably and relax as much as possible. The person is asked to concentrate on the breathing process, preferably through the nostrils, and to lengthen and deepen breathing in and out gradually, evenly and steadily, without hyperventilation. Counting breaths up to 10 and then counting back down to one enables a person to do this easily. The patient is told to try to let the breath come naturally from the bottom of the lungs all the time, that is, by use of the diaphragm.

The technique is often enhanced by instructions to patients to imagine a scene from their life that they associate with feelings of deep relaxation and security. They should focus on relaxing, whilst carrying out the imagery and breathing exercise. The imagery aspect of treatment is designed to divert attention from everyday concerns, from unpleasant thoughts and from pain.

2   *Progressive muscle relaxation (PMR)*. The aim of PMR is to enable patients to become aware of their own muscle tensions and to relax different muscle groups selectively. The

patient should sit or lie comfortably; after a few minutes of abdominal breathing, and starting at the toes, the person should slowly tense and relax the muscles of the foot, followed by those in the calves, thighs, buttocks, abdomen and on up the eyelids; not forgetting the arms and hands. Each muscle group should be tensed for 5 to 7 seconds followed by a relaxation period of 25 to 30 seconds. Concentration on this process tends to eliminate anxiety-provoking thoughts and images from the mind. It is not always possible to complete the whole routine in a busy daily life using the ideal period of 15 to 30 minutes. In such cases, brief relaxation concentrating on specific muscles for 5 to 10 minutes, or even only a few minutes, may bring relief to a painful area. Used in this way, relaxation becomes a habit that is of value in many situations. An important gain from the technique is the ability to distinguish between tense and relaxed muscles. It is important not to tense an already tense muscle, because that would cause additional pain, but instead to use other relaxation skills – see (1) above. A good relaxation technique takes time to acquire and patients may need several practice sessions, and encouragement to continue, if they are to succeed. Occasionally relaxation produces sleep. If this happens regularly, then patients should be advised to carry out the technique when they are not tired. Relaxation is of greatest use in pain that is intermittent and in chronic conditions associated with marked emotional tension. For example, stress-induced headache or back pain often responds well to relaxation techniques.

Hypnosis

Hypnosis is only a short step from an aspect of relaxation therapy, known as guided imagery, in which pleasurable images and scenes are conjured up by patients to distract the mind from tension building thoughts whilst they relax at the same time.

Hypnosis is a process that produces an altered state of mental activity because of susceptibility on the part of the patient, or subject to suggestions made by a hypnotist whether in a clinical or lay setting. Recent experimental work using PET imaging studies has shown that the affective domain of pain, that is the cerebral focus of its emotional element, depends

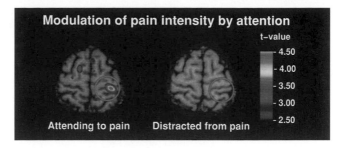

Fig 18.1 PET scan showing regional cerebral bloodflow before and after hypnosis/distraction for the relief of pain. Reproduced from Pain imaging, Progress in pain research and management, Vol 18. IASP Press 2000.

upon activity in the anterior cingulate cortex, whereas the sensory component resides in the sensory cortex. Studies of hypnosis reveal that hypnotic suggestions can be used to modulate the unpleasant quality of pain, or pain intensity. Those changes are reflected in alterations in cortical blood flow in the respective areas. Reduction in the unpleasantness, or intensity of pain, is accompanied by a reduction in cerebral blood flow representing a reduction of brain 'work'. Similarly, with distraction, reduction of cerebral blood flow occurs in the sensory cortex. Therefore, there is evidence now that hypnosis results in an alteration in brain function when pain is being modulated (Fig. 18.1).

Changes in the unpleasant quality of pain, or its intensity, support the observation that hypnotized individuals subjected to pain actually experience less pain as a result of hypnosis rather than merely reporting less pain in response to suggestions. The ease with which hypnosis can be used to reduce or abolish pain varies with the hypnotizability of the individual. Those who are highly hypnotizable show the greatest susceptibility to suggestions made by the hypnotherapist. The common elements of the hypnotic state have been described and are shown in Box 18.3. There is probably a cascade effect from the first to the last condition and that results in the facilitation of suggestions from the therapist, including the suggestion that the pain will lessen. Hypnosis in medical practice is used particularly in dental surgery, or other brief surgical procedures. The use of hypnosis is for those who have been fully trained in medical hypnosis. When pain is chronic, as for example in stress-induced headaches, patients themselves can acquire the ability to use hypnosis in a process known as autohypnosis, which should be taught by a qualified practitioner.

Box 18.3

Elements of the hypnotic state

1   An absorbed and sustained focus of attention on one or few targets.

2   An absence of judging, monitoring and censoring.

3   A suspension of the usual orientation towards time, location and sense of self.

4   The experiencing of one's own responses as automatic (i.e. without deliberation or effort).

5   A feeling of ease or relaxation (manifested as letting go of 'tensions' or becoming at ease, and not necessarily physical relaxation).

From: Hypnosis and suggestion in the treatment of pain by Joseph Barber. Copyright (c)1996 by Joseph Barber. Used by permission of WW Norton & Company, Inc.

Biofeedback

In contrast to relaxation, biofeedback is a systematic approach that involves teaching patients to gain awareness of their physiological responses. This may allow them to achieve a sense of control over those responses to the point where this is achieved without the need for biofeedback equipment.

This process requires a period of training. The therapist monitors one or more selected bodily responses (e.g. muscle tension, surface skin temperature, heart rate or blood flow) and feeds them back to the patient either graphically on a video screen, or auditorily, with the aim of teaching the person to control the visual or auditory feedback. In this way the patient learns to relax muscles, or to reduce their heart rate and their blood pressure. The technique is used to reduce pain in several conditions (e.g. tension headache, migraine headache) using relaxation and thermal biofeedback. The latter technique is used also in individuals with irritable bowel syndrome and Raynaud's disease.

The essence of thermal biofeedback is to teach patients to warm their hands by increasing local blood flow with the assistance of feedback equipment used to monitor the changes. It incorporates a thermometer attached to a heat sensor that registers temperature changes from the skin of as little as 0.1°C. Using a visual trace, or an auditory tone, the patient is encouraged to alter the temperature by mental effort and, surprisingly, this works!

After 8 to 12 sessions of 15 to 20 minutes carried out twice a week, together with 20 minutes' practice a day at home, the individual patient should have learned how to relax and how to alter skin blood flow. There appears to be an overall correlation between satisfactory temperature training and, in the case of chronic tension headache, headache reduction. As might be imagined the use of biofeedback, for whatever purpose, is a matter for experts. Although popular at one time in the United States particularly, biofeedback is not a technique that is used very much in Britain and the more widely adaptable techniques of relaxation and cognitive/behavioural therapy are preferred.

Behaviour modification

This approach to the treatment of chronic pain is based on the knowledge that behaviour, including that associated with pain, is learned. Learning processes may be modified or corrected without necessarily involving direct intervention with the patient's deeper mental life. In other words, if a patient in pain is behaving in such a way that is currently or ultimately disadvantageous in terms of coping effectively with work and interpersonal relationships, then that should be amenable to correction by a system of rewards for 'good behaviour' (adaptive behaviour) and punishments for 'bad behaviour' (maladaptive behaviour). This form of treatment is most effectively carried out in pain management centres by trained staff (usually psychologists or nurses). Patients should attend frequently, or perhaps be resident. In some cases, both modification of behaviour using this method and group psychotherapy are carried out simultaneously.

Fordyce described the principles of this technique in detail in the late 1970s and they are as follows:

1   Behaviour is governed by its consequences. Those consequences that increase the occurrence of a particular form of behaviour are known as 'positive reinforcers' and those that decrease it as 'negative reinforcers'.

2   Behaviour associated with pain can be maintained, enhanced or extinguished by appropriate use of reinforcers. Positive reinforcers include attention, sympathy, concern, rest and analgesic drug administration. Undesirable forms of behaviour (e.g. lying in bed instead of performing some

domestic task, making frequent requests for analgesics or complaining about pain) are dealt with by the withdrawal of positive reinforcers. They are reinstated, if appropriate, only when a desirable pattern of behaviour that has been worked out beforehand has been achieved. In practice this means that desirable forms of behaviour will be noticed, complimented and encouraged (the use of positive reinforcers), whereas undesirable forms of behaviour will be ignored (negative reinforcement), with explanations as to why they have been withdrawn.

Within a relatively short time from the introduction of this form of treatment, that excludes any consideration of mental processes, it was realized that such exclusion was not possible or helpful. As a consequence, a different approach to therapy was developed from cognitive theory leading to the introduction of cognitive/behavioural therapy described in the next section.

Cognitive/behavioural therapy

The psychological basis for cognitive/behavioural therapy for the treatment of pain has been discussed elsewhere (see Ch. 5) and is summarized in Box 18.4. This section describes how these elements may be combined to the benefit of a patient with pain. The four essential components of cognitive/ behavioural therapy summarized in general terms are:

1   Education

2   Skills acquisition

3   Cognitive and behavioural rehearsal

4   Generalization and maintenance.

Education

Having gained the confidence of patients and their relatives, the therapist helps them to alter their perceptions of being able to manage pain and its psychosocial consequences, and also to adjust the carer's perception of the patient's potential ability to improve and to gain control over their symptoms. The therapist encourages both parties to accept that they can learn the skills needed for the patient to cope better with pain and other related problems. These steps are taken to ensure that patients and their relatives fully understand the medical, psychological, social and occupational aspects of the pain problem, and to help them to understand the nature of the

> **Box 18.4**
>
> ## The nature and purpose of cognitive/ behavioural therapy
>
> - Cognitive/behavioural therapy proposes that negative or dysfunctional thoughts influence mood and behaviour.
>
> - The predisposition to think negatively about oneself and illness may have developed in childhood where particular attitudes, including those towards pain and disability, are learned. They may develop also from experiences later in life.
>
> - Cognitive/behavioural therapy aims to help sufferers to view their circumstances more objectively and, as a consequence, feel and behave differently.
>
> - The method of therapy includes education, collaboration, the development of agreed goals, homework and maintaining and evaluating progress.
>
> Adapted from Porter M., Alder, B., Abraham C. Psychology and sociology applied to medicine. Churchill Livingstone, 1999, p.129. Reproduced with permission.

disease or injury and its natural variations. Also, and importantly, the process actually changes cognitions, that is, thoughts and beliefs about pain, its nature, origins and management. On the basis of the work described an acceptable programme is designed with achievable goals set in the context of a 'treatment contract'.

Skills acquisition

This element of therapy is vital and re-establishes lost or neglected skills and behaviour that were part of daily living. Its purpose is to ensure that patients take responsibility for and gain control of their pain. This is achieved usually using imagery and relaxation. The process involves setting behavioural goals for the patient; this reduces reinforcement of pain and disability. The goals include increased mobility, less rest or 'down time', less dependence on medication or the use of mechanical aids such as sticks, crutches or wheelchairs, and an increase in domestic and social activity.

Cognitive and behavioural rehearsal

To establish confidence in patients undergoing a cognitive/ behavioural technique (e.g. relaxation and imagery), it is essential that they should first learn the technique correctly and, secondly, appreciate that the benefits to be gained may take several sessions to emerge fully. Therefore, all individuals will undergo training and repeated rehearsals of the method. They should report back on their success with symptom control, and on any difficulties that they may have encountered in practising the method. In a full programme, the period of treatment may last for 3 months. It may involve the inclusion of relaxation imagery, or possibly biofeedback, from the beginning and the adjustment of goals over time. It is essential that family members should be made fully aware of the techniques being used for goals of the programme, and the need for their involvement and support. In fact, in some programmes, close relatives also learn and participate in the practice of relaxation and imagery in order to give further support to the patient.

Generalization and maintenance

As the programme progresses, usually over 6 to 12 weeks on either an outpatient or inpatient basis, patients and their carers provide reports at weekly intervals on the success or difficulties they have experienced using goal-setting behaviour. Feedback from the patient to the therapist leads to further rehearsal of the changes in perceptions, attitudes and behaviours that are needed to achieve the goals. After a satisfactory period of treatment, success in reaching those goals will encourage further work to consolidate the gains made.

At the termination of active treatment, therapists will seek to generalize the benefits gained more widely to various areas of daily living. They will encourage patients to maintain the gains, by inviting them to make intermittent visits, or regular telephone calls, during which any problems are resolved as far as is possible and successes are reinforced.

It is known that, over time, cognitive/ behavioural therapy will reduce pain, for example in rheumatoid arthritis where mobility increases and emotional problems lessen. It is also known that the effectiveness of the treatment tends to lessen with time if it is not reinforced. Relapses in arthritic patients tend to occur when the patient's symptoms increase in intensity, when the disease process advances, or when the sufferer perceives increased difficulty in retaining control over the symptoms. Their psychological distress increases, and if they abandon the coping mechanisms learned during therapy there is likely to be a major decline in pain control, functional ability and psychological status. Cognitive/ behavioural therapy is widely used by pain practitioners from various professional backgrounds. Those who intend to use it should be adequately trained in its theory and practice. It is used chiefly in chronic pain disorders where complex biopsychosocial problems have developed.

Psychotherapy

Psychotherapy is any form of treatment, including cognitive/behavioural therapy, that is based chiefly upon verbal communication with the patient in contrast to the use of drugs or physical treatment. The techniques to be described are used primarily in psychiatric patients with subacute or chronic pain. Therapy may involve only the patient and the therapist (individual psychotherapy), or it may be conducted with groups of patients who have similar emotional disorders, for example anxiety or anger control (group psychotherapy). If therapy is based upon treatment sessions at frequent intervals, for example daily for 4 days or more each week as in psychoanalysis, it is said to be intensive. It is more usual for patients to attend weekly for 6 to 12 weeks or, at most, 6 months to a year, to undergo brief psychotherapy. The different forms of therapy are outlined below.

Supportive therapy (counselling)

The basis of this form of treatment, summarized in Box 18.5, is that the therapist, who may be a doctor, nurse or other profes-

---

Box 18.5

Counselling

- Counselling requires skills developed through training and practice.
- It can be directive or non-directive.
- It aims to empower people to achieve goals that they choose for themselves.
- It helps people adjust to a new situation or change their behaviour.
- It involves communicating clearly about experiences and feelings.
- It depends upon being able to communicate genuinely and empathetically.
- It involves helping people identify options and to develop plans.
- It has been shown to be effective.

sional, listens carefully to the patient's concerns showing understanding and expressing concern, if appropriate, as the patient is encouraged to put forward conflicts and anxieties. Reassurance and advice are given, and therapists may use their experience in life to help patients to gain a clearer understanding of their own situation. Many doctors in their daily practice when dealing with worried patients who have physical disorders, for example in acute and painful illnesses, use counselling frequently, consciously or otherwise. To share experiences with the patient, therapists need to shed aspects of their professional roles that could interfere with the interaction.

Sharing experiences has to remain under the control of therapists, however, and they must retain emotional integrity especially when dealing with patients' complaints or anger. Therapists must give the impression to patients, both through what is said and their body language (facial expression and body movements) that they have a positive feeling towards them. Often patients express the view that doctors or other professionals do not believe that they have pain, or say that other professionals have implied, or expressed, criticism of their condition. For this reason they may well be very guarded when approached by the therapist and, indeed, may refuse supportive therapy at first. Therefore, from the start a feeling that the therapist is genuine and believes the person to have pain leads to trust. This is crucial in making progress in the therapeutic relationship.

Although special techniques are seldom required when treating acute pain, thoughtful doctors use their understanding of the patient's illness and its effects to gain maximum benefit from the treatment. Acute illnesses result in anxiety and a sense of disorganization for the patient who actively seeks the doctor's support. The patient expects the doctor to be able to restore a sense of orderliness and control by labelling the disorder, describing its course and treatment, by carrying out the treatment, and by giving a prognosis. This provides both a new self-image for the patient and brings the promise of relief. This leads to the collaboration of the patient with the doctor and the establishment of what is known as the 'treatment contract' between them. The purpose of the contract is that the doctor should restore the patient to good health but, being a contract, the doctor expects the patient to be cooperative and make every effort to comply with treatment. Patients who are acutely ill often need to regress, that is to turn from adult to more primitive childish behaviour. They should be allowed to do so as a protective step while in the situation where they are unable to cope alone with the implications of their illness or injury. Such behaviour, though normal, should not be prolonged. By contrast, some patients fail to use this protective mechanism, and continue to carry more responsibility than is good for them once they have become ill.

Following the principles of supportive therapy at an early stage, doctors should give patient a simple factual explanation of the illness, the treatment they intend to carry out, and their expectations about the outcome, being honest about any unpleasant effects the treatment may bring. From time to time, acute disorders lead to permanent changes in the way the body functions, its appearance or to a disability, as for example after bowel surgery where a colostomy is established, after the amputation of a limb, or after mastectomy. Doctors must anticipate the likelihood of such problems, as mourning for the loss of a body part, and prepare patients for it. Patients should never waken from planned surgery to find that a major physical reconstruction, or amputation, has taken place without prior discussion. Patients' relatives suffer disruption of their lives and experience anxieties about the patient's welfare, the future of the family and the problems ahead if long-term medical care or supervision is required. Therefore, they too should be involved in discussions about treatment and its outcome. It is important to remember that difficulties surrounding acute or chronic painful disorders will only emerge if doctors listen, giving patients and their relatives time to express their own feelings, and attempt to understand them.

The success of supportive therapy depends upon helping patients clarify their needs and goals and helping them to develop reasonable strategies for change. This should result in reduced emotional tension and anxiety, lessening of depression and reduction or abolition of maladaptive behaviours. It is essential that both the therapist and the patient understand that the patient has to work towards certain agreed goals, with the help of the therapist. In addition to improvements in emotions, patients should become less reliant on analgesic medication and show less evidence of illness-related behaviour. Finally, therapists need to guide patients away from becoming emotionally dependent on them. Counselling is widely used for the management of physical, psychological and social problems. As with other techniques, it is advised that those who wish to practise counselling should undergo formal training.

Interpretative therapy

This form of therapy is more complex in its structure and more time consuming than supportive therapy. It is carried out by psychiatrists or psychologists who have undergone special training in the techniques involved. It is directed towards helping patients understand the meaning of their symptoms. It involves interpretation of their personal difficulties in everyday life. It requires analysis of the patient's emotional relationship to the therapist, because the former tends to displace on to the latter feelings and ideas that originated in relationships with others. Through analysis of the patient/therapist relationship, and changes that occur in it with time, the significance of varying aspects of earlier emotional events to psychologically determined physical symptoms such as pain may be examined. This form of therapy is occasionally used in those with chronic pain. Patients selected for treatment should have the following general characteristics:

1   An abnormal emotional response to physical illness in terms of its intensity or duration.

2   Pain for which a physical cause cannot be found or that, from the outset, is recognized as being heavily psychologically influenced.

3   Sufficient awareness of their own 'inner mental life' to allow the development of a working relationship with the psychotherapist.

Interpretative therapy is a technique that involves a long period of training and practice to acquire. It is used far less than cognitive/behavioural therapy, relaxation or counselling, and plays a very limited role in the management of chronic pain disorders.

Group therapy

Group therapy, which is sometimes incorporated in pain management programmes, is carried out by a psychologist, psychiatrist or nurse with patients who have pain and, in some instances, with their relatives. The method is economical when several families have relatives in treatment, when it is felt that a patient will have difficulty in establishing a one-to-one relationship with a therapist, or when therapists prefer to let their patients examine and improve their ability to relate normally to others in the presence of those who have similar problems. Other advantages to be gained are that patients' sense of being alone, of being alienated and of being different are reduced in the presence of others with similar physical, emotional and social difficulties. The tendency to emotional dependency on the therapist that develops in one-to-one treatment is reduced. Patients are usually more willing to accept the interpretation of their difficulties and advice about their management from their peers than from a therapist alone. Their fears of serious disease, lifelong difficulties in coping with stresses, problem drug use and other problems can be freely discussed and the group can give support or criticize when appropriate. This adds support to efforts to treat patients outside the group. It helps patients to establish healthy goals that they gradually work towards, thereby obtaining greater satisfaction from work, leisure and personal relationships. Patients are helped to adjust to pain and disability and are prevented from developing unrealistic hopes about recovery and what they will eventually be able to achieve. Preoccupation with themselves may be reduced as a part of developing contact with others.

The purpose of family groups is primarily to educate relatives with regard to the nature of pain and methods used in its control. The psychological and social consequences for both the patient and the relatives are included in discussion sessions. An opportunity for hard-pressed and anxious or angry relatives to exchange feelings with others, to ventilate them and to learn coping skills is usually profitable. Group and family programmes are used chiefly by pain management clinics with teams that include clinical psychologists and nurses trained in psychological methods of treatment.

Conclusions

The methods of treatment described in this chapter should not be seen as simply a matter of applying techniques that 'in themselves' will necessarily lead to recovery. It is important to appreciate that reduction of pain and restoration of function, which results from psychologically based programmes, often removes obstacles to recovery. This means that recovery is possible but first some form of psychological barrier must be removed; a good example is the removal of a fear of pain. For example, this often seriously hampers normal function in those who complain of chronic back pain and disability but with a lack of objective evidence of physical abnormality. A combination of cognitive/behavioural therapy and a programme of graded activity designed to overcome fears and promote activity reduces the level of disability or progression into that state that will otherwise become permanent.

Self-assessment questions

18.1 Which of the following facilitate the effectiveness of clinician/patient communications?

a. Empathy on the part of the clinician
b. The age of the clinician
c. The environment in which the interchange occurs
d. The sex of the clinician
e. Brusque and matter-of-fact behaviour by the clinician

18.2 Which of the following are key elements of cognitive/behavioural therapy?

a. Education
b. Physiotherapy
c. Skills acquisition
d. Fear control
e. Cognitive and behavioural rehearsal

18.3 A 45-year-old woman who is separated from her husband, who drinks to excess and lives with her teenage son who is misbehaving at school, has chronic low back pain. Full investigations by an orthopaedic surgeon and a neurologist have not revealed an obvious physical cause for pain and yet the woman is confined to bed by pain for periods of several days, takes excessive amounts of the narcotic analgesic dihydrocodeine and fails to cope with her housework.

a. What further investigations may be needed?
   i. A further detailed physical examination
   ii. Psychiatric assessment
   iii. Assessment by a multidisciplinary pain management team
b. Which of the following is the most likely diagnosis?
   i. An occult spinal condition
   ii. A somatoform disorder
   iii. A psychosis
c. On the basis of your diagnosis, which of the following treatment approaches is indicated?
   i. Physiotherapy
   ii. Spinal cord stimulation
   iii. Cognitive/behavioural therapy
   iv. Multimodal therapy

Self-assessment answers

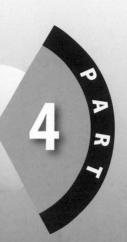

Self-assessment answers

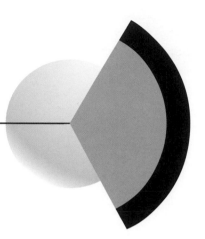

1.1

    a. T

    b. T

    c. F

    d. T

    e. T

2.1 Prevalence: the percentage of individuals in a known population who have the symptoms being studied at some point during a specific time, e.g. 1 month prevalence, 1 year prevalence.

2.2 b, c

2.3 c

2.4

    a. 50%

    b. 90%

2.5 Check your answer against Box 2.3.

Chapter 3

3.1 c, d and e

3.2 VAS, pain drawing and pain diary

Chapter 4

4.1

    a. F
    b. T
    c. T
    d. T
    e. F

4.2

    a. T
    b. T
    c. F
    d. F
    e. T

4.3

    a. T
    b. T
    c. F
    d. F
    e. F

4.4

    a. F
    b. T
    c. T
    d. F
    e. F

Chapter 5

5.1 b, c, e

5.2 a, c, e, f

5.3 a, b, c

5.4 'Burn-out' syndrome

5.5 Refer to Box 5.3.

Chapter 6

6.1

a. T
b. F
c. T
d. T
e. T

6.2

a. F
b. T
c. T
d. T
e. F

6.3

a. F
b. T
c. T

Chapter 7

7.1 a, b, d, e

7.2 a, b, d, e

7.3 b, e

7.4 c

Chapter 8

8.1

a. T
b. F
c. T
d. F

8.2

a. T
b. F
c. T
d. T

8.3

    a.   F

    b.   T

    c.   F

    d.   T

8.4

    a.   T

    b.   T

    c.   T

    d.   F

Chapter 9

9.1

    a.   T

    b.   F

    c.   F

    d.   T

    e.   T

9.2

    a.   T

    b.   F

    c.   F

    d.   T

    e.   F

9.3

    a.   F

    b.   F

    c.   T

    d.   T

Chapter 10

10.1

    a.   3

    b.   4

    c.   1

    d.   5

    e.   2

10.2

    a. F
    b. T
    c. T
    d. F

10.3 c

10.4 c

Chapter 11

11.1 b

11.2 b

11.3 b, c, e

11.4 b, d, e

Chapter 12

12.1

    a. T
    b. T
    c. T
    d. F

12.2 b, c, e, f

Chapter 15

15.1

    a. T
    b. F
    c. T
    d. F
    e. F

15.2

    a. T
    b. T
    c. T
    d. F
    e. T

15.3

    a. T
    b. F
    c. T
    d. F
    e. F

15.4

    a. F
    b. F
    c. F
    d. T
    e. F

15.5

    a. T
    b. F
    c. T
    d. F
    e. F

15.6

    a. F
    b. T
    c. F
    d. F
    e. T

15.7

    a. T
    b. F
    c. F
    d. T
    e. T

15.8

    a. T
    b. T
    c. F
    d. T
    e. F

15.9 b

16.1

a. T
b. F
c. F
d. F
e. T

16.2

a. T
b. T
c. F
d. F
e. F

16.3

a. F
b. T
c. F
d. T
e. F

16.4

a. T
b. F
c. F
d. F
e. T

16.5

a. F
b. F
c. T
d. F
e. T

17.1

a. F
b. T
c. F
d. F
e. T

17.2

    a. F
    b. F
    c. F
    d. T
    e. F

17.3

    a. F
    b. T
    c. F
    d. T
    e. F

17.4

    a. F
    b. T
    c. F
    d. F
    e. F

17.5

    a. F
    b. F
    c. T
    d. F
    e. T

Chapter 18

18.1   a, c, d – in some cases

18.2   a, c, e

18.3

    a. iii
    b. ii
    c. iv

Index

Please note that references to non-textual information such as Boxes, Figures or Tables are in *italic* print

G

H

U